✓ The first step in treatment consists of putting the patient on an anti-yeast diet such as the one outlined in this book.

✓ The next step usually entails restoring the affected mucose membranes and skin to a healthy condition.

✓ The third step is the control of the Candida overgrowth, which involves taking a fungistatic preparation.

✓ The final step in managing Candida involves using agents like acidophilus and other friendly bacteria.

✓ In addition to close adherence to the diet and the program outlined, a cleanup program of the patient's environment, usually carried out under the supervision of a health professional, is extremely important.

SILENT MENACE

Twentieth Century Epidemic—
Candidiasis

Dorothy Senerchia

with Introduction, Case Histories, and Afterword
by Andrew L. Rubman, N.D.

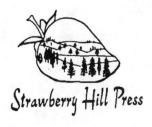

Strawberry Hill Press

Copyright © 1990 by Dorothy Senerchia

Strawberry Hill Press
2594 15th Avenue
San Francisco, California 94127

Edited by Sara Shopkow

Proofread by Catherine J. Nichols

Back cover photo by Adriana

Cover by Ku, Fu-sheng

Designed and typeset by Cragmont Publications, Oakland, California

Printed by Edwards Brothers, Inc., Lillington, North Carolina

Manufactured in the United States of America

Library of Congress Cataloging-in-Publication Data

Senerchia, Dorothy.
    Silent menace: twentieth century epidemic—candidiasis / by Dorothy Senerchia ; with introduction, case histories, and commentary by Andrew L. Rubman.
        p.   cm.
    Includes bibliographical references (p.)
    ISBN 0-89407-094-0 : $9.95
    1. Candidiasis—Diet therapy.   I. Rubman, Andrew L.   II. Title.
RC123.C3S46   1990   89-27646
616.9'69—dc20   CIP
                                                       AC

DEDICATION

This book is dedicated to the memory of
Gladys Regier Vaughan
in gratitude for her knowledge, her influence, her
once-in-a-lifetime friendship, and her enduring inspiration.

SPECIAL THANKS

To my mother, Theresa Senerchia, for her loving support, patience, and untiring assistance during the many hours I spent developing my recipes in her wonderful kitchen in Warwick, Rhode Island.

To Doctor Andrew L. Rubman, for his professional help with editing the medical content of the book and for providing the Introduction, Afterword, and case histories of patients of the Southbury Clinic in Southbury, Connecticut.

To my editor, Sara Shopkow, for lending her expertise, dedication, and total commitment to the book.

To my publisher, for offering me the opportunity to get this information to the multitude of Candida patients who need it.

And to two special sisters, the true midwives of this book, for lending their knowledge as health writers, their experience in the world of publishing, and their extraordinary support from the day they saw my first outline. There are no words that express my gratitude to Lydia Wilen and Joan Wilen.

Acknowledgments and Special Thanks to:

James A. O'Shea, M.D.
Janet Mariani
Noëlle Brisson
Carmen Tagle
Timothy Gray
Ana Martinez
Paul Roebling
Martha Danielle
Lucy Petrarca
Wellington S. Tichenor, M.D.
Gladys Vaughan
Anthony P. Galzarano, D.C.
Stella Adler
Susan Simon
George F. Kroker, M.D.
Jessy Pierre-Louis
Ruth Beaufays
Teresa Laughlin
Michelle Russell
Ellen Lohsen
Don Reis
Christina Senerchia
Adriana Kleiman
Jacqueline Ceballos
Bette Henritze
Fabio della Sala
Manon Brady
Jennifer Longrée

Table of Contents

Introduction

This book will serve as an inspiration to the many who suffer from vulnerability to the yeast organism *Candida albicans*. Rather than presenting a rehash of the staid diets of those many books that have gone before, Dorothy Senerchia incorporates her knowledge of international cuisine into a book that makes Candida dieting and everyday survival a palatable lifestyle for the Candida patient. She not only proves it is possible to work, socialize, travel, and function in the mainstream of life, while adhering to a highly restrictive diet and treatment program, she presents it as a joyful experience.

As a Candida patient who has taken a positive approach to her own problem, the author transmits her optimism, allowing her readers a more open and self-confident perspective and a more positive attitude toward the world around them.

I urge all those who feel they may be vulnerable to Candida or who may care about someone who suffers from it, to keep this book in a prominent place in the household. It is a valuable reference and a comfort to those who have to restructure their diets to restore a compromised immune system.

Andrew L. Rubman, N.D.

Preface

In January of 1980, I developed arthritis in my right knee. I had a number of other discomforts, including itchiness all over my body, and thighs that were swollen most of the time. I became more and more tired and less able to walk around on a debilitated knee. No doctor could give me an explanation.

Two years later, after developing a headache which lasted many weeks, I was sent for a CAT scan to investigate the possibility of a brain tumor. When I was injected with the iodine dye used for this type of test, I had a severe allergic reaction, manifesting itself in swollen eyes, intolerable itching all over my body, and a dangerous swelling in my throat.

The CAT scan revealed no problems. However, at a later date, I recounted the iodine dye episode to a medical assistant at Mount Sinai Hospital in New York City who suggested I look into the possibility of other allergies. As a result, I got skin tests from a traditional allergist which revealed that I was highly allergic to many foods. After several days of eliminating the offending foods, I experienced tremendous improvement in my symptoms, but there was still plenty of unexplained discomfort, including in the troubled knee (which by that time had been subjected to what was probably an unnecessary operation). It took another two full years before I found out that my allergic propensity was related to an abnormal yeast growth called *Candida albicans*.

In the spring of 1984, after returning from a gastronomic binge in Paris, what I would now call a "yeast feast," I went to see an allergist-nutritionist whose lab I had been frequenting for periodic tests for food allergies. I was not only having allergic reactions to more and more foods, my right elbow was in pain and my entire right arm had stiffened to an almost ninety-degree angle. Fortunately, by that time I was sophisticated enough to know that joint pains could be food related, so I sought help from an allergist rather than from my orthopedic surgeon, who found my symptoms more baffling than I did.

After looking at my elbow, making note of the skin rashes on my feet and hands, and asking me several questions, the allergist said he had a hunch as to what might be causing both the stiff arm and the increasing number of food allergies. He gave me a copy of *The Yeast Connection* by Dr. William Crook, asked me to read it, and to come back and tell him if the problems discussed in the book "rang any bells for me."

I spent the greater part of the next weekend riveted to the book because a great deal of it sounded familiar. What happened between the day I finished the book and started the Candida control diet and the birth of renewed vitality, is history. When I go home now, my mother tells me my personality has changed, that I am more like my younger self, full of energy and enthusiasm. I am so different from the woman who used to collapse on the couch after breakfast. I realize now that the itching that plagued me, and the need to lie down after breakfast, were part and parcel of an allergic reaction to the wheat, coffee, and milk I ate every morning. I always knew the arthritis in my knee went hand-in-hand with the itching in my thighs, but every doctor to whom I told this only listened and responded with a mystified look. It wasn't until I went on the Candida control diet outlined in Dr. Crook's book and eliminated the foods I'm allergic to that I discovered I didn't have to put up with my arthritis. As the pains in my joints disappeared and my right arm slowly unstiffened, a myriad of other discomforts also left me. I am a renewed person, and for that reason I have decided to share what I've learned with other people.

In the pages that follow, I have tried to explain what *Candida albicans* is and described in detail the diet which alleviates its many symptoms. Since I'm an experienced cook, I have included a section on cooking techniques which are necessary to follow the Candida diet successfully, and a collection of recipes which I originated myself or adapted to the Candida method of preparing food.

I offer the book not only in the hope of helping those people who may have arthritis related to *Candida albicans*, but also to provide an avenue of investigation for those who are plagued with other symptoms for which they can find no explanation.

CHAPTER ONE

Candida Albicans

What Is *Candida Albicans*?

Some people think *Candida albicans* is an opera singer. Would that it gave us so much pleasure! This much talked about yeast organism, which keeps a low profile in the bodies of all of us, can get out of control and multiply when given the opportunity. If and when such multiplication occurs and *Candida albicans* becomes aggressive and compromises the mucous membranes of the body, toxic by-products may enter the bloodstream, creating a condition called "atypical" or "chronic candidiasis" (which I will call "candidiasis"), as well as the potential for a whole host of symptoms.

A person who has a systemic yeast infection or "Candida," as the illness is commonly referred to, can become excessively fatigued, depressed, irritable, or all three. While the yeast problem is more characteristic of women, men also find themselves prone to the viral and bacterial infections, intestinal gas, constipation and/or diarrhea, psoriasis, athlete's foot, and migraine headaches which often go hand-in-hand with Candida. Suffering from joint pains, sexual impotence, or a loss of concentration is very common. Partial loss of hearing or deafness, declining vision, Premenstrual Syndrome, frequent urination, or a combination of any number of the above symptoms, are frequently found in the Candida patient. Many people who have the problem crave desserts, candy, starchy foods, dairy products, and alcohol. They may feel bad on damp days and in moldy places, and many develop multiple allergies as well as an inordinate sensitivity to chemicals and cigarette smoke.

An important factor to be considered in diagnosing Candida is that most of the discomforts mentioned above can also be symptoms of other illnesses. For that reason, the patient should be given a comprehensive medical examination and a full battery of tests at the outset to rule out the possibility of other illnesses. If all the tests show negative results and the symptoms persist, it behooves the doctor to investigate the possibility of candidiasis. A common scenario with Candida patients is as follows: One develops the symptoms (but not the actual condition) of a recognizable illness like reactive hypoglycemia, a low blood sugar disorder. The physician, unaware that the symptoms are secondary to candidiasis, treats them accordingly, leaving the root cause, the yeast infection, unattended and free to generate other complications.

How It Happens

There are millions of people who have undiagnosed candidiasis. One of the most common ways of developing the illness is by using the popular broad spectrum antibiotics known as Tetracycline, Keflex, Ceclor, ampicillin, amoxicillin, Septra, and Bactrim. The intestinal flora, so vital to our health, sometimes called "friendly bacteria," are injured by the drugs in the course of their attack on the harmful bacteria. When drug treatment is over, the lack of normal intestinal bacteria allows *Candida albicans,* previously kept in check, to multiply into large families and "colonize" on the mucous membranes of the gastrointestinal tract and, in the cases of women, in the vagina as well.

The arrival of the new Candida colonies signals the beginning of trouble because the immune system, the complex mechanism which defends our bodies and fights off disease, is unduly challenged by the overgrowth of *Candida albicans* and is no longer able to keep the Candida under control. The Candida then produces toxins which are released into the system, giving rise to a myriad of symptoms. To put it simply, *antibiotics suppress friendly bacteria, allowing yeast to multiply. Yeast produces toxins and toxins generate symptoms.* The body, as a consequence, becomes immunologically taxed and much more prone to illness.

Let's take the example of a woman who took antibiotics on several occasions and, weakened by an overgrowth of yeast, develops a viral infection. Unaware of what drugs have done to her body, she goes to an established doctor who diagnoses her virus accurately but *prescribes an antibiotic which, while necessary for controlling a bacterial infection, is not necessary in the case of a viral infection.* She takes the drug, feels better for a while, and discovers later that she's more debilitated than ever. Why? Because the unnecessary antibiotic the doctor gave her has taxed her immune system even further. It's a repetition, in fact, of what caused her to become prone to developing a virus in the first place. *This is the vicious cycle of Candida.*

It should be made clear here that when a Candida patient develops a *bacterial infection,* which has been identified by a proper culture, and an antibiotic must be taken, his or her doctor should be consulted regarding the degree to which the anti-yeast medication should be increased. Patient and doctor should also discuss the kind of intestinal bacteria (like acidophilus) to be used to strengthen the friendly flora in the intestinal tract, which have been compromised by the antibiotic.

Use of steroids, such as cortisone or prednisone, for bursitis or other rheumatic ailments, also produces a pattern of Candida overgrowth in some people. A woman in my family is a case in point. Periodically she suffers from arthritis in her right knee and gets a cortisone shot because it makes her feel better. The shot eventually takes its toll because the steroids weaken her immune system. The pain she was initially trying to alleviate comes back because the underlying problem hasn't been addressed.

There's a close relationship between the body's hormonal balance and yeast. Birth control pills contain progesterone and upset the hormonal balance in some women. Increased progesterone, as exists in the case of pregnancy, promotes vulnerability to candidiasis because progesterone facilitates the overgrowth of yeast. Incidentally, newborns who acquire *Candida albicans* during the birth process are often more susceptible to Candida infection later on.

A Modern Illness

In the nineteenth century when people still rode in a horse and buggy, they were exposed only to certain chemical by-products in the form of fumes from candles and gas lamps, the combustion of paper and chemically-treated tobacco in cigar and cigarette smoke, and an occasional fire that swept the town. Their systems reacted, but since the incidence of toxic exposure was far less frequent for them, their systems adjusted. The pollutants they breathed added up to a drop in a large barrel compared to today.

The state of weakened immunity seems to be related to the twentieth century. I have a friend who has Candida and has said on a number of occasions that he's "allergic to the twentieth century." His description of it as an allergy to this era is certainly on target.

In the course of one day in twentieth century America, we're exposed to exhaust from vehicles; pollution generated by industrial facilities and jet engines; impurities in drinking water; additives in food; smoke from tobacco, marijuana, and charcoal broiling; chemical cleaning agents; fumes from dry cleaning; gas from the kitchen stove; formaldehyde, polyurethane, shellac, nail polish, pesticides, fertilizers, and weed killers; chemical odors generated by synthetic carpeting and fabrics; gases from petroleum products like wax and plastic; and the lead in paint. The rain that falls on us and everything we eat, drink, or inhale is polluted! Our immune systems and our bodies, which are challenged from all sides, weren't designed to handle the twentieth century overload.

Add to an already over-taxed system a dietary intake of refined flour and food that's been so over-processed it's lost many of the vitamins, minerals, and nutrients needed to maintain a strong immune system. Combine that with a high intake of refined sugar, which diminishes the effectiveness of the white blood cells needed to combat disease, and it's amazing any of us are still walking around!

Adelle Davis, in *Let's Eat Right to Keep Fit,* said that when food shortages in World War I prompted the government of Denmark to forbid the processing of grains, nutrition improved so markedly that not only did the incidence of cancer, diabetes, high blood pressure, and heart and kidney disease all take a sizeable drop, the death rate fell thirty-four percent!

Have you thought about the fact that with all the progress in medical research and modern medicine, widespread epidemics of incurable illness are more threatening than ever? We hear of one terminal case after another. Yet the discussion and speculation about the great mystery surrounding these epidemics continues. The only mystery, it seems to me, is why enlightened public officials and legislators, who are in a position to do something about the pervasive health problems of today, are so few and far between.

Getting Help

It's been said that it takes society a hundred years to move an inch. This is certainly true of the medical profession vis-à-vis the role of *Candida albicans* in human illness. When Dr. C. Orian Truss of Birmingham, Alabama first began to speak about Candida more than twenty years ago, he found few listeners. And even today, after publication of his substantive and enduring book, *The Missing Diagnosis,* the idea of Candida as a possible link in the web of certain complex medical problems such as rheumatoid arthritis, osteoarthritis, multiple sclerosis, migraine headaches, premenstrual syndrome, lupus, cystitis, Crohn's disease (inflammation of the intestine), sexual impotence, chronic depression, and schizophrenia is still met with profound resistance from the majority of established doctors. It's heartbreaking to think how many more people will become prone to serious illness before the medical establishment loses its resistance. Fortunately, there are some doctors who've been willing to incorporate Dr. Truss's research into their practices, to the great advantage of their patients.

In diagnosing Candida, the doctor relies heavily on "clinical suspicion," looking at the medical history of the patient and the patient's family, the presenting symptoms, the history of drugs taken in relation to the time of the onset of symptoms, and the patient's answers to certain crucial questions like "When did you last feel well?" The goal of treatment is to restore the immune system so it can regain its former ability to keep *Candida albicans* under control.

If you think you have Candida, the most effective way to proceed is to try to locate a health professional with knowledge of the immunological problems associated with *Candida albicans* overgrowth. If you can't find a knowledgeable doctor, go with one who is understanding and willing to research the subject. A cooperative immunologist or naturopath could provide a plan of diagnosis and treatment, and in some towns there are nutritionists who know how to treat Candida.

The problems of multiple allergies, weight control, hormonal imbalance, and psychological symptoms often associated with Candida must be addressed after the yeast is under control. The usual procedure in managing Candida overgrowth includes a blood test, specifically, a serological test known as an anti-Candida antibody assay. The most effective one in use is the test developed by Dr. Edward Winger of the Immunodiagnostic Laboratory in San Leandro, California. After test results are interpreted, a treatment program is begun.

The first step in treatment consists of putting the patient on an anti-yeast diet such as the one outlined in this book. The next step usually entails restoring the affected mucous membranes and skin to a healthy condition. This can be accomplished with anti-oxidants (such as vitamins and minerals) and products designed to restore normal environment, such as bulking agents, buffering salts, and moisturizing preparations. The third step is the control of the Candida overgrowth, which involves taking a fungistatic preparation such as Capricin, Micocydin, or Paracan. Nystatin, Ketaconazole, and other synthetics are coming into question by some doctors because of the strain these drugs put on the system. The process of controlling Candida overgrowth is often the most difficult step, since the killing off of Candida releases the same toxins into the system that are liberated during its period of overgrowth. Because of this, a slow and steady introduction of the fungistats usually produces the best results. The final step in managing Candida overgrowth involves using agents, like acidophilus and other friendly bacteria. These should restore a normal environment in the intestine so that if the remaining Candida should try to take over again, it's suppressed by an environment similar to the one that held it in check before the problem began.

In addition to close adherence to the diet and the program just outlined, the total cleanup of the patient's environment (his or her rooms, car, and place of employment) and the minimizing of any exposure to molds, dust, perfumes, smoke, and other chemical by-products are extremely important. A cleanup program of this nature is usually carried out by the patient under the supervision of a health professional or as explained in books which are available in health food stores.

Candida very often goes hand-in-hand with multiple allergies. This very important subject is discussed in the next chapter.

CHAPTER TWO

Allergy

If I told you that sometimes I get up in the morning feeling good and then go off to work walking with a limp after having a couple of slices of toast, would you believe me? While it's true that I have a fertile imagination, this has happened too many times for me to think it's all in my head. I dragged a painful knee around for more than two years without the remotest idea it was related to what I ate.

If you so much as suspect you have candidiasis, you should have allergy tests, which include foods, inhalants, and chemicals. The presence of allergy in Candida patients is very common and you may be experiencing symptoms directly related to foods you eat or to something in your home like synthetic fabrics, dust, mold, fumes from the garage, or any number of things around you. From the way I understand it, the toxic by-products of *Candida albicans* overgrowth can penetrate the body's intestinal wall and enter the bloodstream, increasing allergic sensitivity. In many cases, Candida can create the potential for *multiple* allergies. A person with one or two allergies may or may not have Candida, but a person with many allergies should, by all means, investigate the possibility. The relationship between Candida and allergies is one of the areas in which doctors who treat Candida have a lot more to learn.

What Is Allergy?

Being allergic means that you react abnormally to a substance to which most people don't react at all. Having an allergic reaction to an egg is a good example. What could be more basic to the life process than an egg? Inhalants like timothy grass and the pollens in the air are natural and harmless and most people don't react to them. When our white blood cells produce certain proteins, called "antibodies," against normal substances (in wheat or in oranges, for example) called "antigens," we know that our immune system is engaging in allergic reaction. When the antibodies and antigens interact, complex symptoms may appear, many of which may be recognizable as allergic symptoms.

Allergies can affect any organ of the body. Among the more common symptoms of allergy are stomach distress, itching, joint stiffness or pain, fatigue, nausea, sore throat, coughing, sinusitis, pressure in the chest, heart palpitations, earaches, itchy ears, ringing in the ears, and hives. Even the brain can be affected. The toxins producing an allergic reaction and those generated by such a reaction, are carried to the brain via its ample blood supply. These toxins can affect the neurons of the brain and give rise to sudden moodiness, irritability, outbursts of temper, depression, hyperactivity, and other symptoms commonly regarded as psychogenic.

Continuing to eat and breathe allergens can weaken the immune system. I mentioned earlier that, at one time, my arm stiffened to a ninety-degree angle. I had gone to Paris and lived it up on cheese, bread, wine, and sweets. Not only was I knowingly eating foods to which I was allergic but, unbeknownst to me, I was nourishing the *Candida albicans* already out of control in my system. Although I was in a wonderful frame of mind in Paris, I developed a cold, sore throat, and sinusitis which I couldn't get rid of. At one point I stopped my allergenic foods for three days and started to feel better. As soon as I resumed the wine, cognac, bread, and sweets, my immune system weakened again and the cold and other symptoms returned.

For two weeks after the trip, I walked around New York in a daze, confused when crossing the street, forgetting my belongings on the way to work, and generally disoriented. There was pain in my arm and elbow. After further indulgence in food and wine, my arm slowly began to stiffen. I didn't know what was happening at the time. I know now that it was Candida plus allergy at work.

Do You Have Allergies?

Most people will say "no" when asked if they're allergic to anything they eat or breathe. However, since some experts say that more than thirty million Americans have allergies, it wouldn't be surprising to find out that you're one of them. Given the number of new chemicals and pollutants introduced into our foods and environment giving us the potential for developing allergies, it would seem reasonable for you to take a look at how your own body functions. You could start by asking yourself some of these questions:

- ☐ Are you troubled with postnasal drip, sinusitis, and frequent sore throats?
- ☐ Do you often feel very tired after waking up from a full night's sleep?
- ☐ Do you frequently feel exhausted, bloated, or have excessive gas after a meal? Do you burp long after you've finished eating or between meals? Does your body retain a great deal of fluid?
- ☐ Are there specific foods or beverages you crave? Are there any you feel you couldn't live without, like coffee, popcorn, chocolate, dairy or wheat products?
- ☐ Are there any foods to which you have an adverse reaction, even the day after eating them?
- ☐ Does a moderate amount of wine, beer, or any other alcoholic beverage make you feel bad? Do you get a hangover from one drink?
- ☐ Do you ever feel like you have a hangover after you've had food but no alcohol?
- ☐ Do you have a pallid facial color and/or dark circles under your eyes? Are your eyelids often swollen?
- ☐ Did you have epilepsy or asthma as a child? Were you hyperactive?
- ☐ Does the presence of cats, dogs, or horses bother you even when they're not active?
- ☐ Do perfumes, certain soaps, toothpaste, or body powders bother you?
- ☐ Do you often feel depressed or irritable for no reason at all?
- ☐ Do any members of your family, including grandparents, aunts, or uncles have asthma or hay fever? Do any of them appear to have addictions to alcohol, drugs, sugar, or other foods? Do they suffer from headaches, arthritis, or stomach problems?

If you answer "yes" to even two of the above questions, you should suspect that you have allergies and you should arrange for an evaluation. There are so many people walking around with undiagnosed symptoms who refuse to even entertain the idea that their symptoms might be related to allergy. You don't want to be one of them.

Testing for Allergy

Allergy testing presents problems because most of the testing methods have a low rate of accuracy. However, some of them can be useful. Here are some of the tests your health practitioner may suggest:

The *Radio-Allergo-Sorbant Test (RAST)* uses a blood sample to test the amount of immunoglobulin E (IgE) and immunoglobulin G (IgG) present for specific foods and inhalants. The test can yield information regarding both immediate and delayed reactions caused by foods. Some doctors feel this is the most reliable test for allergies, providing a very competent laboratory is used. One of the better laboratories I know of that provides analysis of RAST testing is the Alletess Laboratory in Rockland, Massachusetts.

The *provocative test method* consists of injecting a small amount of the suspected substance (the antigen) under the skin. If an inflamed circle, a wheal, appears around the area of injection, it's an indication of allergy. The size of the wheal will give some indication of the degree of allergic sensitivity after a waiting period of ten minutes or so. These tests, which yield more accurate results on some people than others, are also employed in determining the dosage to be used in injections for desensitization to inhalants, a common and often successful form of immunotherapy considered very helpful by some Candida patients.

Sublingual testing can be administered by a doctor simply by placing a tiny drop of extract from various foods, chemicals, pollens, dusts, and molds underneath the tongue. An allergic individual may develop symptoms within minutes with just a few drops of the extract. The response may parallel the allergic reaction the individual would have if in contact with the allergen itself in a conventional, everyday environment. Some doctors find sublingual testing very useful.

Cytotoxic testing, not yet available in every city, must be carried out by highly-trained technicians. This method is used more for testing for food allergies than for chemical or drug allergies. The purpose of the test is to indicate whether or not certain changes occur in the individual's blood cell appearance, which some physicians feel is indicative of sensitivity to antigens in the foods being tested.

The procedure requires that the test foods be eaten during the two week period before the test. Each of the suspect foods is mixed with a sample of the individual's white blood cells from freshly drawn blood and added to a culture of blood components. There's a sensitivity scale of one to four; the person tested may get a three on veal and only a one on banana, suggesting that there's only a slight allergy to banana. Along with the problem of a low accuracy rate, the extract used in cytotoxic testing often contains chemicals, which the patient may react to rather than to the food being tested. Nevertheless, some patients find cytotoxic testing helpful.

Kinesiology is another allergy testing method currently in use. The underlying principle here is that what affects one part of the body may affect the other parts. Muscle strength is established before the test and after the food being tested is ingested, the muscle is retested immediately. If there is a lack of resistance in the muscle when it's retested, this is a possible indication of allergy. A certain amount of controversy surrounds this method of testing.

The *traditional scratch test*, administered on the skin, produces inaccurate results approximately eighty percent of the time. For this reason, the test is no longer used by most modern allergists.

Testing Yourself for Food Allergies

You can try food allergy testing on your own with the help of a professional. One common method is through use of the elimination diet. Start by making a list of all the foods you eat on a regular basis like eggs, milk, wheat, corn, sugar, oranges, etc. Then make sure you eliminate these foods for seven days, after which you'll begin to fast. In this way, you'll free yourself of any symptoms that may be evoked by having these foods in your system. And, if and when any symptoms arise following reintroduction of a suspected food during the test, any confusion about which foods are responsible will be eliminated.

The recommended way of using the elimination diet method is to go on a fast *supervised by a knowledgeable health professional* for approximately five days. This is *not* something you should do on your own. You should arrange your life so that your activities are curtailed during the fast, since you'll probably have less energy than usual.

Begin by eliminating everything but sea salt and spring water sold in a glass bottle. (Plastic provokes a reaction in some individuals.) Don't worry about dying from starvation. There are people who fast for up to three weeks and there have been cases of people lost far from civilization who went without food for more than double that amount of time and survived. You may feel hungry at the beginning of the fast, but that will only last for a day or two; at a certain point your body will begin to draw upon its own reserves. You may experience withdrawal symptoms on the second or third day of fasting when the body begins to notice the lack of foods it's accustomed to. Resist the temptation to eat!

At the end of the fast period, start introducing, *one food at a time,* the foods you eliminated during the seven days before the fast. Eat no more than one food for breakfast, such as diluted orange juice (nothing hard to digest), one for lunch, like a baked potato, and one for dinner, like fish. Try not to overindulge yourself. Needless to say, seasoning these foods in any way could complicate the test. Cooking brown rice with chicken broth or broiling scallops with safflower oil, fresh dill, and lemon might cause allergic reactions to the added foods. You wouldn't know if you were reacting to the foods you want to test or to the added foods. It's also important to consider avoiding foods wrapped in plastic packages sealed with heat, because the food may have absorbed chemical fumes from the heated plastic. If you're sensitive, you may react to the chemicals rather than to the foods you're testing.

Everything used in food testing must be as pure as possible. To test for rye, for example, buy rye crackers with no yeast in them (Wasa Lite Rye, Finn Crisp Light Rye, Ryvita Light Rye, or Floridor). To test for yeast, use the Red Star brand, which is free of corn. (Empty one packet or the equivalent amount of yeast into a glass of ice cold spring water or fresh fruit juice, if you already know you don't react to the juice.) People who have Candida are supposed to stay away from chocolate because of its dairy protein and sugar content, but if you want to do a chocolate test anyway, use Baker's Unsweetened Chocolate to be sure any reaction is to the chocolate and not to the sugar. Nuts used for testing should be very fresh so you won't be reacting to any mold they may have acquired. You can toast them in the oven if you like.

The process of reintroducing previously eliminated foods should be done slowly and one at a time. It could be handled something like this:

Day One
    Breakfast: diluted orange juice
    Lunch: baked potato
    Dinner: fish
Day Two
    Breakfast: banana
    Lunch: carrots
    Dinner: chicken
Day Three
    Breakfast: egg yolks (do egg white on another day)
    Lunch: broccoli
    Dinner: brown rice
Day Four
    Breakfast: grapefruit
    Lunch: string beans
    Dinner: lamb

Do this until you've tested yourself for all the foods you eliminated previously and any other foods you suspect might be causing allergic reactions. Ten days of testing in this fashion should be the maximum. A reasonable portion of each food should suffice; remember your body isn't used to large meals at this point. If, for any reason, you feel you must repeat some of these foods, let a four-day interval elapse before repeating them.

Allergic Reaction

If you have an allergic reaction during this process and want to attempt to counteract it immediately, take two level tablespoons of baking soda and one level tablespoon of potassium bicarbonate (from the drugstore) and thoroughly mix them. Add the mixture to two cups of tap or spring water and drink.

Another simple way to counteract allergic reaction is to use a packet of Alka Seltzer Gold tablets (not to be confused with Alka Seltzer). (Be aware that these tablets are very high in sodium and should be sanctioned by your doctor.) In about eight ounces of water, mix one of the two Alka Seltzer Gold tablets contained in the packet and drink. Dissolve the second tablet in another eight ounces of water and drink. When doing this in a restaurant, you shouldn't be tempted to settle for a single tablet because there's only one glass of water on the table. However, if that second glass of water is too difficult to get, the one tablet will go far in helping you to feel better. I've taken Alka Seltzer Gold many times without the awareness of anyone at the table. Here's how these wonder salts work: There are local acids that accumulate at the sites where reactions are occurring; the salts buffer those acids and normalize the body's chemistry very quickly, alleviating the symptoms.

Eliminating Allergens

The most effective way to avoid allergic reactions is to eliminate the foods that provoke them. If cow's milk gives you symptoms, eat foods that are free of cow's milk. There are some wonderful allergy cookbooks on the market which contain a number of milk-free recipes. I've developed some good milk-free muffins and quickbreads which are in the recipe section. (Remember to eat them sparingly because they're high in carbohydrates.)

If you're one of the many people who react to the protein in cow's milk *rather than the lactose* (milk sugar), you can try drinking and cooking with goat's milk (in either fresh or powdered form) which doesn't contain the beta lactoglobulin (a common allergy provoking protein) found in cow's milk.

Goat's milk is also more healthy. One reason is that goats aren't injected with potentially harmful hormones and antibiotics as are cows. On many dairy farms in the United States, cows with leukemia or other illnesses are still milked, as well as processed for meat! (In Europe, they kill all cows that have diseases, no matter how large the number.)

To successfully avoid eating allergens, you have to know all the likely and unlikely places they can be found. This involves serious detective work. Wheat, for example, can be found in many more places than you might imagine. You might expect to find wheat in pasta, crackers, matzo, pizza, pretzels, breads of most kinds, waffles, and pastries. But would you think to look for wheat in meat loaf, canned soups, luncheon meats (including salami), soy sauce, MSG (monosodium glutamate), malt (most malt is made with barley), or alcoholic beverages (whiskey, vodka, and beer)?

Here's an example of the pervasiveness of wheat. One night I visited a couple who had prepared beef stew for dinner. Since they'd been very considerate and checked out all the ingredients in the stew with me in order to avoid any allergens, I felt quite comfortable about eating it. However, as it turned out, I developed a headache during the evening and the next day I awakened feeling exhausted. My eyelids were heavy, as they often are the day after I've eaten allergenic foods. I was amazed to react that way because I'd so carefully avoided the French bread, ice cream, and wine and asked for lemon and oil on my salad (to avoid vinegar). But later, as I mentally reconstructed the conversation about the dinner, I remembered the host and hostess saying they'd used an old family recipe that required adding Bisto to the stew. A few days later, I found Bisto in the supermarket and lo and behold, one of the ingredients listed on the package was wheat!

Corn is another good example of a common allergen that's found in more places than you might expect. You may know you're eating corn when you eat popcorn, tortilla chips, cornstarch, and corn flakes. But corn can also be found in frankfurters, certain margarines, some commercial baby foods, some canned soups, some malts, whiskey, bourbon, gin, and beer. A lot of sugar products, like confectioners sugar, dextrose, glucose, and some commercial syrups, contain corn. Whiskey, bourbon, gin, and beer can also contain corn.

Corn can be found in body powders, soaps, and some toothpastes. Equal®, the low calorie sweetener, contains "dextrose with dried corn syrup." Manufacturers modify their recipes from time to time but, presently, such products as Campbell's Cream of Mushroom Soup, Cool Whip, and Green Giant Frozen Spinach Soufflé all contain corn in some form. Who would have thought that instant coffee and the glue on postage stamps contain corn? The cornstarch in baking powder is something to be aware of since so many recipes call for baking powder. (You can avoid the corn by making your own baking powder with an arrowroot or potato starch base. See the recipe in this book.)

If you find that you have food allergies, you should be aware that acquiring more allergies is very easy. This can happen by eating the same foods over and over. How many times a week do you eat chicken, beef, potatoes, or eggs? Frequently, I'm sure. This is a pattern that should be reversed if you have food allergies. If you want to get rid of an allergy you've already identified, try eliminating the food in question from your diet for two to six months and you may lose your allergy. However, if the allergy doesn't go away after such a long abstinence, it could mean that you have a fixed allergy, one that you were born with that will linger on.

Dr. Herbert Rinkel developed a highly useful method of rotating foods called the Rotary Diversified Diet. This system, sometimes referred to by slightly different names, involves eating all foods on a four-day rotating schedule and can be very helpful in preventing individuals who have food allergies from developing more of them. Because knowledge of this method is so important for people with allergies, I've covered the rotating system in another chapter.

For those of you who know you have food allergies, I should inject a word of caution here. Make sure you chew your food very well. If you don't, you run the risk of not having it properly digested. Bacteria in the large intestine acting on undigested food may produce substances that provoke allergic reaction.

I should reiterate that you should avoid inhalants that trigger reactions in you because they, too, further the growth of Candida. Staying away from cigarette smoke or smoke from any source, is very important. If you live in a city and ride the bus, avoid sitting next to a highly perfumed woman, if perfume bothers you. When crossing the street, wait for the bus to pass and let the pollution rise into the air before you walk to the other side.

In summing up, try not to deceive yourself about the importance of identifying what you're allergic to. Commit yourself to staying away from your allergens. I know people who avoid yeast, sugar, and fermented foods religiously and still feel bad a great deal of the time. It's hard to convince them that staying on a Candida diet and rotating foods are not going to do much good if they're constantly assaulting their immune systems with food and inhalant allergens. *Eating and breathing what you're allergic to weakens the immune system and a weak immune system can't keep* Candida albicans *under control.* Hopefully, after treatment, the many allergy problems induced by Candida will be greatly minimized or will possibly disappear.

CHAPTER THREE

The Candida Diet

Some people will tell you you're in for a very rigid program on the Candida diet. Actually what may seem like a rigorous and arduous regimen in the beginning will become second nature after a while. I know a number of people who've been on the diet for an extended time. Many of them make breakfast for the family, get to work, go out to restaurants, parties, movies, and the theater. In short, they're thriving people, functioning in the mainstream.

The Candida diet brings many benefits with it. It reduces the amount of unnecessary starch intake and, for some, makes the loss of weight automatic. It encourages you to feed your system the much needed nutrients found in foods that are unprocessed and free from chemicals. Those of you who choose to follow the rotating diet will also have your gastronomic horizons expanded because you'll be eating from a very varied menu to eliminate repetition. Converting to this new way of eating, free of sugar, chemicals, and additives, will probably lift your spirits as well as improve the quality of your skin and hair. Many people have told me I look much younger since I've been on the Candida diet.

I'm sure you've been told that being on an anti-Candida regimen entails a great deal of deprivation. Let me make your day by telling you how many superb treats you're in for. Delectable dinners of beef, lamb, and chicken with succulent vegetables, sausage meat for breakfast (depending on your cholesterol considerations), pasta in moderation, and a bun-less hamburger with lettuce and tomato are all on the diet. Broiled, baked, or fried fish are on the menu along with mussels, little neck clams, shrimp, scallops, lobster, and caviar. Also included are omelets, salads galore, and vegetables of every shape and color. Just a few of the treats on the snack menu are zucchini sticks, guacamole and tortilla chips, nuts, yeast-free crackers with almond, sunflower or sesame butter, and potato chips. Once in a while you can even have small portions of homemade jello, pancakes, cookies, and other delights which you'll find in the recipe section of this book.

You're going to be able to eat out as well as entertain at home. Your daily regimen will feature fresh vegetables and foods high in protein rather than carbohydrates. What the diet requires is a shift in some of your cooking and eating patterns, and planning ahead. Instead of peanuts and pistachios, you'll be eating walnuts, almonds, hazelnuts, pecans, pine nuts, and brazil nuts. Rather than unselectively taking oil from the grocery shelf, you'll make the shift to looking for cold-pressed vegetable and nut oils.

A Preview of the Candida Diet

Bearing in mind that the basic principles of the Candida diet are discussed in greater detail in the chapter entitled "The Principles and Techniques of Candida Cooking," here's a preliminary explanation of how to proceed during the initial months of dieting.

Essentially the foods to stay away from are yeast, sugar, vinegar, and fermented substances like apple cider (fresh apple juice is not a problem), aged cheese, and soy sauce. Molds, yeasts, and products of fermentation are all cousins and should be avoided.

Most Candida diets prohibit mushrooms and related fungi like truffles and Chinese tree ears, but since it's been found that most people don't have trouble with mushrooms and since they're used in so many recipes, you should try having them and see how you fare. If you do well with mushrooms, they'll give you some potassium and selenium, enhance your soup stocks, and add gourmet panache to your dinners.

Nuts, a great source of fiber, are included in the diet. They tend to acquire mold when sitting in a shop for a long time, so look for the very fresh, raw, unprocessed nuts. Toast them if you like, but not to the point of drying out the oils in them.

Dried spices and herbs can be used freely when heated long enough to kill any mold. In uncooked dishes like salads, use only fresh herbs. Fresh mint, dill, parsley, basil, tarragon, chives, and sage will add a great deal of flavor to both cooked and uncooked dishes. A dinner of roast lamb with dill gravy, accompanied by a baked potato smothered with fresh chives and a large, ripe, garden tomato baked with a topping of fresh basil, will please both you and the family. Fresh herbs are also healthier than dried herbs which, in most cases, are irradiated to extend shelf life. You can grow herbs easily in your garden or on your window sill. If you can't find the plants locally, some of the large mail order nurseries or companies like Williams-Sonoma will ship them.

Instead of using salad dressings containing vinegar or sugar, you should have oil with lemon, lime, or orange juice on your salads. Check the recipe section for new salad dressing ideas or come up with some of your own. Commercial mayonnaise contains vinegar, sugar, and preservatives but, as you'll see, making your own is a simple matter and you'll probably love the results. Soy sauce, which is fermented, is a no-no, but Chinese food without soy sauce is very good. A platter of shrimp with crunchy snow peas, bean sprouts, fresh ginger, garlic, and salt sautéed in oil, for example, is first rate.

Eating aged cheeses (they're fermented) won't be helpful. Roquefort, because of its high mold content, is considered the least desirable. Some health professionals will tell you to stay away from the fresh, unfermented cheeses too. Others will say that cottage cheese, cream cheese, farmers cheese, ricotta, mozzarella, and fresh goat cheeses are okay, even though they're made with a bacterial culture. It would be a good idea to talk this matter over with your doctor. Whether or not you should have yogurt, sour cream, buttermilk and crème fraîche should also be discussed.

Tofu is allowed on the Candida diet. Miso isn't, because it's fermented. If you don't react adversely to it, butter is okay, but margarine, a synthetic product, is not recommended. Any product whose list of ingredients contains the words "whey," "casein," or "caseinate," has cow's milk in it and should be avoided if you're allergic to cow's milk.

As for sugar, there are many sweeteners to be avoided. Refined and unrefined sugar (sucrose) top the list. You should also abstain from glucose, maltose, lactose, sorbitol, corn syrup, maple syrup, date sugar, molasses, and honey. The controversial saccharin and aspartame (NutraSweet®) are also on the list. Intake of fructose, the natural sugar contained in fruit and fruit juice, will have to be limited for some people and avoided altogether for others. Some health practitioners insist that all fruits are off limits, while others say you may have them once in a while, depending on the extent that fructose stimulates the growth of yeast in you. I suggest that you look for your own level of tolerance. If you have to limit your quota of fruit, the best way to proceed might be to have a half fruit before your meal. Be very mindful of how much fructose you can handle when using fruit and fruit juice to sweeten your muffins, quickbreads, pastries, and other desserts. If you've concluded that you should eliminate fruit entirely, make muffins without chopped fruit and use plain water instead of fruit juice. (This works especially well with the muffins I've developed using Fearn Rice Baking Mix.)

Raisins, dried apricots, dates, prunes, and figs have been through a drying process and may contain sulfites; they also may have formed mold. In addition, they're high in natural sugar, so if you can't resist them, use them in very small amounts. But make sure they're heated for at least ten minutes to kill any mold. As you'll see, dried fruit is added sparingly to the dessert recipes.

Wine, cognac, beer, vodka, gin, scotch, rum, liqueurs, and other fermented beverages like apple cider are off limits. Alcoholic drinks are not only fermented, they're made with brewer's yeast; many of them, like wine, also contain chemicals, mold, and sugar. Hopefully, you won't be without them forever. I have an occasional glass of wine or champagne now that my Candida is under control.

Foods containing malt such as malted drinks and certain cereals and crackers should be avoided too. Hopefully, manufacturers will market more products free of malt and yeast as consumers begin to ask for them.

Freshly squeezed juices like orange, grapefruit, apple, carrot, beet, and whatever else may be available at the coffee shop or juice bar are allowed, depending on how much natural sugar you can handle. Bottled and frozen juices should be boiled first if you're super sensitive to mold. Seltzer water, club soda, and bottled mineral waters are fine. You can make good drinks by adding a few squirts of fresh berry, citrus, or other fruit juice to seltzer water. "Pink Champagne" made with pureèd red watermelon (see recipes) is also recommended. Strong Cranberry Cove tea (an herb tea made by Celestial Seasonings), iced, with a small amount of vitamin C crystals (ascorbic acid) added, is a fine substitute for wine at dinner.

Drinking herb tea is preferable to coffee and normal tea because the latter two involve a drying process and usually contain mold. For that reason, you should skip them for now. This is also true of instant and brewed decaffeinated coffee and tea. Taheebo tea (Pau d'Arco), said to have anti-fungal properties, is highly recommended. It comes in bulk and in tea bag form and can be found in health food stores. If you feel that you can't start the day without coffee, try decreasing your intake and see how you feel.

Bread and bread crumbs contain baker's yeast, the yeast that makes a loaf of bread so airy and puffy. Fortunately, there are yeast-free crackers like Carr's Table Water Biscuits, matzo, Ryvita Light Rye, and Wasa Lite Rye, all of which can be found in supermarkets. Rice cakes (large puffed brown rice wafers), brown rice crackers (made by Westbrae, Robata Snacks, Hol*Grain, Edwards & Son, and others), and white rice crackers (by Ka-Me and Ono) are all good to eat. You should stay away from crackers made with soy sauce or tamari (they're fermented). If you're industrious, you can make your own crackers out of a variety of unenriched flours.

Some commercial cakes, pastries, and other raised baked goods also contain baker's yeast, but you can make your own by using baking powder or baking soda. Many pie crusts have neither sugar nor yeast in them. As long as the fillings are made of something that doesn't contain sugar or the other sweeteners previously mentioned, you can make delicious turnovers, pies, and pie crust rolls. When trying to determine whether or not freshly baked goods have sugar or yeast in them, phrase your question judiciously. If you ask: "Does the flour in these pastries contain yeast?" the salesperson might very well say "No." If you ask: "What ingredients are used in these pastries?" you'll probably get a more accurate answer from the salesperson, who won't know what you're trying to avoid. Some salespeople will answer honestly no matter how you phrase the question, bless them. As you'll see in the recipes, it's quite easy to make your own pastries and muffins using natural sweeteners; some of them can be made in batches for freezing, a great way to save time.

Smoked products like salami, frankfurters, pepperoni, and most of the commercially marketed sausages tend to acquire mold. They also usually contain dextrose, corn syrup, sugar, and a variety of preservatives, including the much talked about sodium nitrite, which can induce degenerative changes associated with cancer. These foods are not recommended. Fortunately, fresh sausage, free of sweeteners and chemicals, is becoming more available. I would highly recommend the chemical-free sausages made by Schaller & Weber in New York City. They're shipped to other places around the country in sealed bags which allow them to stay fresh for a longer period. One delightful sausage they make, weisswurst, contains veal, pork, and seasonings;

its taste resembles that of a frankfurter, but weisswurst is free of the ground bone and cornmeal fillers often found in commercial frankfurters. Schaller & Weber also make a bratwurst of pure pork and seasonings. There's also an excellent Italian sausage called "Papa Cantella" which is chemical-free and found in supermarkets. If you can't find a product that's free of chemicals and sugar, try having your local sausagemaker make one to order.

A Word About Supplements

Since your consumption of dairy products is curtailed on the Candida diet, you should resolve what to do about your calcium intake with your doctor. Women over thirty-five, including those who don't have Candida, should take calcium supplements. This may help to avoid osteoporosis (loss of normal bony tissue resulting in brittle bones). Bear in mind that, if your body lacks calcium, it will start drawing calcium from your bones. Vitamin D is needed to absorb most dietary calcium, so individuals who have little or no exposure to direct sunlight or who have some other problem that prevents adequate synthesis of vitamin D, may need to take it as a supplement. This should be done under supervision, since vitamin D is potentially the most dangerous of all vitamins if taken in excessive doses.

There are a variety of calcium supplements available on the market. Some, such as Nucalmag, a calcium/magnesium butyrate, are almost entirely absorbed, regardless of the problems connected with normal mineral absorption characteristic of some Candida patients. Others, like the carbonates and amino acid chelates, are best absorbed when taken with citrus fruit, if you've determined that you can have fruit. This should be worked out with the person who's treating you.

Green vegetables, soybeans, sardines with bones in them, salmon, oysters, almonds, hazelnuts, and sunflower seeds are all good sources of calcium. You can make delicious salads by combining some of these foods with ripe tomatoes, cucumbers, radishes, fresh herbs, and a vinaigrette dressing of lemon or lime juice, or mayonnaise.

I'm not suggesting that you take calcium or calcium plus vitamin D supplements by themselves. You need a good multiple vitamin and mineral supplement containing sufficient vitamin A (recommended by your doctor) as well as additional vitamin E, vitamin C, and zinc to help boost the immune system. If you have a high chemical sensitivity, you may want to take a selenium supplement too, but this should also be yeast-free and done only with doctor's approval. Because supplements should be geared to each individual's needs, this is something you should work out with your own health professional.

In keeping with the yeast-free lifestyle, it's also important to remember, when taking vitamins, that many low potency B-Complex vitamins are derived from yeast. You must check all bottles to make sure your vitamins are free of yeast, sugar, and starch. For those with food allergies, special vitamins free of corn, soy, wheat, yeast, sugar, and other possible allergens are available in health food stores and in some drugstores. There's no point in dieting diligently if you're ingesting ingredients contained in your vitamins that encourage the growth of Candida.

Summing Up

Be aware that the program I've just outlined is primarily intended for the initial months on the diet. As you improve, you can experiment with adding more complex carbohydrates, more fruits and fruit sugar, and some of the other foods you've curtailed or eliminated. I know people who've been able to add apple cider vinegar and baker's yeast to their diets after a while and who've done quite well. Only you and your medical adviser can resolve how your diet should be modified.

It's important to understand that *proteins don't nourish Candida albicans.* You can fare rather well if your diet features fowl and game, meat, fish, shellfish, and eggs, as well as salads, vegetables, tofu, unrefined vegetable oils (excluding corn oil), and nuts (except peanuts and pistachios). Whole grains and legumes are also important but must be eaten in smaller portions because of their high carbohydrate content.

Since you'll be on a different regimen and you won't know how it will affect you, you should ask your doctor to check your cholesterol and uric acid levels from time to time. Some individuals on a Candida diet have a tendency to eat too much meat, eggs, and nuts, elevating their cholesterol intake. Please be mindful of this. Until the diet becomes second nature to you, the following lists of what you should and should not eat can be used when shopping for food or eating in a restaurant. Be aware that these lists are intended to provide general guidelines for a diet that must be tailored to meet the specific needs of each person.

Foods Allowed

Applesauce, unsweetened
Arrowroot starch
Baking powder
Baking soda
Butter
Cheeses, fresh (with doctor's approval): cottage, cream, *chevre frais* and Montrachet (fresh goat cheese), farmers, mozzarella, processed American, ricotta
Clams
Cocoa, unsweetened
Coconut, unsweetened
Cornstarch
Crab, canned or fresh
Crackers, yeast-free
Custard, sugar-free
Diet sodas (occasionally)
Eggs
Fish, canned, not smoked
Fish, fresh or frozen
Fructose (fruit sugar) in small amounts
Fruit in measured amounts, if allowed at all
Fruit juice, fresh, in small amounts
Grains, enriched and unmilled: amaranth, brown rice, buckwheat, corn, millet, oats, quinoa, rye, wehani rice, wheat, white rice, wild rice

Foods Not Allowed

Alcoholic beverages
Allergenic foods
Bacon
Beer, alcoholic *and* non-alcoholic
Black bean sauce
Breads with yeast
Buttermilk
Canadian bacon
Candy
Charcoal broiled foods
Cheeses, fermented
Chili sauce
Chinese mustard
Chocolate
Chocolate drinks
Cocktail sauce
Cocoa, sweetened
Coconut, sweetened
Coffee
Corn oil
Corn solids
Corn syrup
Custard, frozen
Dextrose
Duck sauce
Enriched flour
Frozen yogurt
Fruit, canned in syrup
Fruit, dried and uncooked
Fruit juice, bottled or frozen
Ham
Herbs, dried, if uncooked
Honey
Horseradish sauce

Foods Allowed

Heavy cream, without added
   sugar
Herb tea
Herbs, fresh
Herbs, dried (cooked)
Mayonnaise, sugar- and
   vinegar-free
Meat, except smoked
Meatballs (homemade only)
Meat loaf (homemade only)
Milk, cow's and goat's, in small
   amounts
Mineral water
Muffins (homemade)
Mushrooms
Mussels
Nut butters, except peanut
Nut oils
Nuts, except peanuts and
   pistachios
Oils, vegetable (except corn)
   and nut
Pasta, in limited amounts
Popcorn, chemical-free, in
   small amounts
Potato chips, chemical-free, in
   small amounts
Potato starch
Quickbreads (homemade)
Salt
Sausage, fresh (not smoked),
   without additives
Seltzer water
Sesame butter
Shellfish, canned or fresh, not
   smoked
Soda water
Spices, dried (cooked)
Sunflower butter
Tapioca
Tea, herb and Japanese green

Foods Not Allowed

Ice cream
Ice milk
Jams and jellies
Ketchup
Malt
Maple sugar and syrup
Mayonnaise, commercial
Molasses
Mustard
Pastry, commercial
Peanuts
Peking duck sauce
Pepper relish
Pickles
Pistachio nuts
Plum sauce
Puddings
Sausage, dried or with additives
Sherbet and sorbet
Sorbitol
Smoked products: fish, game,
   meats, poultry, shellfish
Spices, dried and uncooked
Sugar (sucrose)
Tea, except herb and Japanese
   green tea
Turbinado sugar
Vinegar
Yeast, baker's and brewer's

Foods Allowed

Tofu

Tortilla chips, chemical-free, in
small amounts

Vegetable oils (except corn),
unrefined and
cholesterol-free

Vegetables, bottled,
chemical-free

Vegetables, fresh or frozen,
preferably low-carbohydrate

CHAPTER FOUR

The Principles and Techniques of Candida Cooking

Candida cooking doesn't involve a totally new method of preparing food; it entails making a few ingredient substitutions and some adjustments in preparation. These adjustments also apply to certain popular ethnic cuisines such as Italian, Mexican, Chinese, and French. The following list of basic principles of Candida cooking will be discussed in this chapter:

☐ Eliminate rot and mold before cleaning and cooking food.
☐ Eat dried spices only if cooked.
☐ Use natural sweeteners only.
☐ Keep carbohydrates to a minimum.
☐ Eliminate alcoholic beverages and products containing alcohol.
☐ Use milk minimally.
☐ Use leavening agents other than yeast.
☐ Avoid products containing malt.
☐ Eliminate vinegar, and pickled and fermented foods.
☐ Substitute fresh meats and fish for smoked products.
☐ Use dried fruits sparingly.
☐ Use unrefined, unsaturated vegetable oils or butter.
☐ Select unenriched, stone ground, unmilled flours.
☐ Use fresh or frozen, rather than canned ingredients.
☐ Avoid chemicals, additives, and preservatives.
☐ Eliminate peanuts and pistachios.
☐ Maintain a hygienic kitchen and refrigerator.

Eliminate Rot and Mold Before Cleaning and Cooking Food

Some fruits, like pears and apples, have a protective coating of yeast. The foggy whiteness on grapes is yeast, too. Also, fruit has usually been sprayed with pesticides. For both these reasons, fruit should be thoroughly washed and wiped dry *whether or not you plan to peel it.*

Wash fruit, as you would your own hands, with a bar of mild soap and warm-to-hot water. After washing and rinsing, dry the fruit with a towel and rub as if polishing it; this should rid the skin of any undesirable coatings. You can wash fruit with any mild soap you're not allergic to. I use a pure olive oil soap made in Greece, which I get in health food stores. It's very mild, made from a natural source, and agrees with my skin. Sandalwood soap is another possibility.

Fruit readily acquires rot. Remove this with a sharp paring knife. Strawberries, a good example of fruit that rots rapidly, should be washed thoroughly in cold water and the rot trimmed just before serving.

Non-leafy salad vegetables like cucumbers, carrots, and radishes should be washed with soap and water and rinsed before cutting. Whenever possible, peel and cut them just before serving to avoid losing nutrients.

Peppers and tomatoes are a different matter because they're often covered with a wax coating to insure freshness after traveling long distances (i.e. from California to the east coast). It's amazing that the state of California allows this practice, since it's now common knowledge that ingesting wax can induce cancer. To remove the wax-coated skin from a tomato, put it on the end of a fork and hold it in boiling water until the skin is soft enough to be peeled off with a paring knife or with your fingers. As for waxed cucumbers or yellow turnips (rutabagas), you can peel off the skin with a knife or a vegetable peeler. This applies to waxed fruits as well.

Melons are not recommended for two reasons: One, they have a high natural sugar content (especially red watermelon); two, mold very often forms on their skins. The melon least recommended is cantaloupe because its porous skin often allows mold to penetrate into the melon. Now comes the "however": If you *must* have melon once in a while, look for one without mold. Wash the skin with soap and water and rinse and dry it just as you would an apple or pear. When cutting a melon, be mindful that as you cut, mold from the skin can accumulate on the knife and travel into the flesh. On those occasions when I have melon for dessert, I rinse and wipe the knife as I peel off the skin.

Are you ready for the Chlorox® bath? There's a doctor in Massachusetts who recommends washing vegetables, including leafy ones, with Chlorox® to eliminate mold. This process is explained in *The Yeast Connection* as follows: Using a stainless steel measuring spoon, measure ½ teaspoon of Chlorox® for each gallon of water used. Place fruits and vegetables in the bath and soak them for fifteen minutes. In the case of fruits and vegetables with heavy skins, soak them for twenty minutes. Timing is essential with Chlorox® bathing. Remove foods from the bath and soak them for an additional fifteen minutes in fresh, clean water, using new water for each batch of food. Dry them and place them in bags for the fridge or freezer. Food keeps longer and mold contamination is minimized when this process is used.

When heating leftovers, which collect mold quickly, cook them for ten minutes at high heat to kill any invisible mold. If you have a stew from four days ago that you're ready to eat again (using the concept of the rotating diet), you should heat it for at least ten minutes so that mold and bacteria won't be a problem. If you can actually see the mold, get rid of the food altogether. Accumulating mold and letting mold spores pervade the refrigerator are not advisable.

Eat Dried Spices Only If Cooked

Dried spices and herbs are likely to acquire mold and should only be eaten if they're used in food that's been boiled, broiled, or roasted at 350° for at least ten minutes. Whether you're using dried rosemary in a stew, curry powder in a sauce, or a cinnamon stick in stewing fruit, you should make sure that these dried herbs or spices are cooked at high heat for ten full minutes. If you're heating up broth from another meal and you want to add a new dried spice or herb, make sure the broth containing the new dried seasoning boils for ten minutes. (If you're using fresh herbs, that won't be necessary.)

When using dried herbs and spices, pour them into your hand or into a cup first, away from the cooking pot; then add them to the preparation in the pot. To pour them directly out of a jar into a steaming pot allows moisture to enter the jar and possibly form mold.

Use Natural Sweeteners Only

As mentioned before, all sweeteners must be eliminated except for those that are totally natural, like unsweetened fruit and fruit juice. Frozen concentrated juices, like orange, apple, and pineapple, can be used as long as they're unsweetened and cooked at high heat (as when used in baking muffins). White grape juice, which usually comes in a bottle, is a very good sweetener, but it should be used sparingly because of its high natural sugar content. In addition, it usually contains mold, so boil it first if it isn't going to be used in a cooked dish. Welch's, After The Fall, and other companies make white grape juice. I often use Lehr's, a brand imported from Germany.

Ripe bananas, pears, peaches, blueberries (watch for mold), or bottled sugarless applesauce can also serve as sweeteners. When I use chopped apple, as I do in some muffin recipes, I usually use a McIntosh; it's sweeter than most apples. It can be too runny for an apple turnover, so use a yellow Delicious apple for that. You can make a wonderful fruit sauce out of canned, sugarless, crushed pineapple in its own juice thickened with arrowroot starch, but do boil both the pineapple and juice for ten minutes since they come from a can. This fruit sauce has plenty of natural sugar and should be doled out in small portions to yourself and guests who are on a Candida diet. Using it on roast duck gives the bird a whole new personality.

Cinnamon and nutmeg can also be used to lend sweetness and flavor, but they're dried spices and should be cooked before you use them. Unsweetened coconut shreds can be added to pastries and salads for added sweetness. Stay away from amazake, a liquid made from brown rice, found in health food stores. It sweetens food admirably, *but it's fermented.*

It's easy to get carried away with natural sweeteners and I must caution you again that fruit and fruit juices should be used minimally. Fruit sugar (fructose), although more easily used by the body than refined sugar (sucrose), nourishes Candida too. The amount you include in your diet should be discussed with the health professional treating you.

Keep Carbohydrates to a Minimum

Since carbohydrates behave like sugar in relation to Candida, by all means keep them at a minimum. Some health professionals feel that the first month of Candida dieting should be as free of carbohydrates as possible, so discuss this with whoever is treating you and plan your diet accordingly. Those of you who are taking an anti-fungal agent should be aware that there's no point in attacking yeast with medication if you're feeding it food that's high in carbohydrates. Many patients deceive themselves in this area.

If you're planning a day's meal, remember that one-half gram of complex carbohydrates per pound of body weight per day is a good measure. For example, a person who weighs 150 pounds should consider 75 grams of carbohydrates a good place to stop. Also remember that complex carbohydrates, those found in whole grains, vegetables, and legumes, are more desirable than the simple carbohydrates found in white rice and white (refined) flour. Whole wheat pasta is better for you than white pasta. In any case, when eating any pasta, including Chinese rice vermicelli, be mindful of carbohydrate grams. Get yourself a carbohydrate counter at a bookstore or a health food store, or such government publications as handbooks numbers 8 and 456 from the U.S. Department of Agriculture. You'll be amazed at the carbohydrate content of some foods: A large grapefruit, usually touted as one of the great diet foods, has thirty grams of carbohydrate, while four ounces of pine nuts have only thirteen grams. If you're developing your own recipes and want to know the carbohydrate gram count per portion, add up the total number of carbohydrate grams for all ingredients used in the recipe and divide by the number of portions you would serve to get the carbohydrate count for one portion.

The gluten-containing grains (barley, oats, wheat, and rye) feed yeast more than the gluten-free grains (rice, buckwheat, millet, and soy), so feature the latter in your cooking when you can. It's also advisable to be tested for a gluten intolerance before selecting grains for your meals.

How often should you eat muffins, quickbreads, cookies, and pancakes made according to Candida guidelines? Eventually you'll know how much rice you can eat, how many chick peas you can add to the soup or the salad, how many crackers you should spread your sunflower seed butter on, and how often you can have muffins or pancakes for breakfast. Hopefully, your intake of carbohydrates can be increased as you begin to feel better.

Eliminate Alcoholic Beverages and Products Containing Alcohol

Cooking with wine, cognac, rum, or other alcoholic beverages is *off limits*. Lemon juice, plain or diluted with water, can sometimes be used as a wine substitute; try experimenting on the side with a small amount of sauce rather than risking an entire potful. Alcohol is found in extracts like vanilla, so try to find pure vanilla extract or use the vanilla bean itself. You can pulverize the bean in the blender if you want a powdered form of vanilla. As for recipes that call for beer in the batter, try substituting club soda.

Use Milk Minimally

Milk should be used as little as possible. It contains its own sugar (lactose) which nourishes Candida. In addition, a large number of individuals have a lactose intolerance. Many people react to beta lactoglobulin, an allergy-provoking protein in cow's milk, and should use goat's milk instead. Remember that goat's milk contains milk sugar too, and should also be used sparingly.

You can use heavy cream or butter in cooking, but know that there's some beta lactoglobulin in the milky solids. Whenever possible, clarifying butter, that is melting it to separate the fat from the milky solids, is the best idea. Be aware that you can use water or *unsweetened* soybean milk as a substitute for milk in some recipes.

Use Leavening Agents Other Than Yeast

Baking will seem limited without yeast, at first, but you'll learn to get a rise out of baking powder. There are many recipes that require baking powder, baking soda, or both. You can make rye bread, soy bread, and many types of biscuits using baking powder. Apple, pumpkin, and carrot breads (called "quickbreads" because they have no yeast) can be mildly sweetened with mashed fruit or fruit juice instead of with sugar or honey.

If you react to corn, which is used in the baking powder one normally buys, make your own baking powder according to the recipe in the recipe section. Or you can use the corn-free baking powder (Featherweight makes it) sold in some health food stores, providing you pay attention to the directions on the bottle. The amount required will differ from conventional baking powder. See to it that the baking powder you have on hand is fresh, because no baking powder keeps its fizz forever. Try to find baking powder that's free of aluminum.

You may crave bread in the early days of dieting, but you'll adjust to having a few yeast-free, whole grain crackers as a substitute. They're high in carbohydrates, so have all crackers in moderation. Breaded foods are often served in restaurants and should be avoided because bread crumbs contain yeast.

You can still have southern fried chicken and fried zucchini sticks, as long as you make some adjustments in the preparation. In cooking at home, you can substitute wheat bran, oat bran, matzo meal, or blender-pulverized rolled oats or barley flakes (found in health food stores) for conventional breading. Ryvita or Wasa Lite Rye crackers, sesame seeds, sunflower or sesame meal, finely-ground nuts, or a batter made of beaten egg and yeast-free flour can also be used as replacements.

Avoid Products Containing Malt

Malt, which is sprouted grain, may be processed from yeast-fermented barley, corn, or wheat and may contain maltose, a close relative of sugar. It's sometimes found in crackers and is almost always found in cereals like puffed rice and puffed wheat, including most varieties found in health food stores. Avoid these products, and remember that certain companies like El Molino and Barbara's Bakery make cereals without malt which are also available in health food stores.

Eliminate Vinegar, and Pickled and Fermented Foods

There are many, many fermented foods used in contemporary cooking, such as vinegar, soy sauce, tamari, and miso. There are also a number of commercially-marketed foods which contain pickled and fermented ingredients. Among these are green olives, sauerkraut, relishes, pickles, horseradish, ketchup, and gravy enhancers such as Kitchen Bouquet® and Gravy Master®.

Commercial mayonnaise contains vinegar, but you can make your own using fresh lemon or lime juice (see recipes). Lemon or lime mayonnaise will get rave reviews in your chicken, turkey, crab, and lobster salads. Adding a small clove of raw garlic or some shallots, fresh herbs like tarragon, basil, dill, chives, or scallion tops, when the mayonnaise is still in the blender or in the beating process, gives it even more flavor. Lemon or lime mayonnaise can be used as a dip for raw vegetables, or for chips and crackers that are considered "legal" on the diet. Adding avocado and/or three or so anchovies, or tuna, crab, salmon, clams, or sardines to homemade mayonnaise also makes an interesting dip.

As for cheese, eliminate the fermented cheeses entirely and bear in mind that even the fresh, unfermented cheeses are made with a bacterial culture that can feed yeast. Also note that, with the exception of those made from goat's milk, cheeses may contain beta lactoglobulin (a protein found in cow's milk) to which you may be allergic.

Let me reiterate that fresh cheeses should be avoided too, unless your doctor specifically tells you it's all right to have farmers, cottage, cream, and fresh goat cheese. Processed cheese (like the one used on most commercial hamburgers) and mozzarella (including buffalo milk mozzarella, which is imported from Italy) are considered fresh cheeses too.

Substitute Fresh Meats and Fish for Smoked Products

Bacon, ham, bologna, salami, luncheon meat, corned beef, and pastrami are smoked, as are many sausages and some turkey. In most cases, these foods also contain chemicals and dextrose. Fresh sausage and frozen, unsmoked sausage that is chemical-free (as are some of the sausages bearing the brand name of Jones), are allowed. If you can't find fresh sausage in your town, you can buy ground pork or veal and season it with sage, marjoram, and some of the other herbs traditionally used in sausage.

There are some French-style patés (check the contents) which are also allowed. Some patés contain wheat flour, to which you may react, and many patés contain truffles, which are fungi to which some of you may be sensitive. The most trouble-free paté is the one you make yourself (see "Country Paté" in recipe section).

Charcoal broiling entails smoke and chemical by-products that encourage yeast overgrowth. Cooking food in the oven or in the broiler of the kitchen stove and bringing it out to the terrace or back yard is preferable. Since commercial barbecue sauce usually contains sugar and vinegar, try basting chicken or meat with lemon or lime and herbs, or sprinkle spices like curry and chili powder on them before cooking. Fresh garlic and/or shallots can be rubbed on the meat or used in a marinade.

Use Dried Fruits Sparingly

As mentioned previously, dried fruit, such as figs, papaya, pineapple, apricots, dates, raisins, pears, peaches, and apples may contain sulfites and may have formed mold during the drying process. They should be eliminated altogether, or consumed in very small amounts, providing they're boiled first. (I've never cooked dried papaya so don't hold me responsible!) If you put a few raisins (very few, I hope) in your cookies here and there, they will bake at high heat in the cookie dough. Raisins, like other dried fruit, are high in natural sugar content, so don't use them until you're familiar with your level of tolerance for fructose.

Use Unrefined, Unsaturated Vegetable Oils or Butter

Your diet should feature unrefined or pure cold-pressed oils that have not been heat-treated. They should also be rich in polyunsaturates and free of preservatives and cholesterol. Erewhon, Hain, Spectrum, and other companies make them. Use these oils in salads, cooking, and baking, and store them in the fridge.

If you're rotating foods, you'll need to have at least four different oils on hand. Olive, soybean, safflower, and sunflower oils are some with which you may already be familiar. Linseed, walnut, almond, pecan, apricot kernel, avocado, sesame, and cottonseed oils, though less common, are good choices too. You can find some of these oils in the supermarket and most of them in health food stores. Olive oil, you should know, contains oleic acid, which is helpful in combating Candida. Soybean oil is highly recommended by some people. Corn oil is not recommended, because it breaks down into arachidonic acid, which can promote inflammation.

Select Unenriched, Stone Ground, Unmilled Flours

Enriched flour usually contains yeast and, in the process of being refined, has been robbed of many necessary nutrients. Unfortunately, in many states in the U.S., there are laws requiring flour, baking mixes, and baked goods to be enriched if sold to the public. Hopefully, you can find a health food store which sells the wonderful stone ground, unenriched flours packaged by Arrowhead Mills, Elam, and Featherweight, among others. You'll especially appreciate the great variety of flour offered by these manufacturers if you're allergic to wheat. Sprouted grains are highly recommended if your health food store has them.

Store flour in the fridge or, better yet, the freezer, if you don't use it regularly. At room temperature, both the vitamin E and flavor in flour can be destroyed. Fearn Baking Mixes, found in health food stores, are highly recommended. There are some good recipes on the sides of the Fearn boxes that can be adapted for your use. I've developed several recipes which are in this book, using their brown and white rice baking mixes, including a real treat called "Candida Pizza." The various types of unenriched, unmilled flour mentioned above can also be used to coat cutlets and vegetables when frying or baking them, since these flours don't contain yeast.

Use Fresh Or Frozen, Rather Than Canned Ingredients

Canned foods should be avoided whenever possible because they sometimes contain mold and chemicals. Even when they don't, the can itself is usually lined with plastic or phenolic compound, which can provoke a reaction in some people. Before opening cans, be sure to wash the tops with soap and hot water and wipe them dry. This is to remove dirt, dust, insect debris, and whatever else might have accumulated there. Frozen ingredients are quite acceptable if free of chemicals. Bottled foods are preferable to items packed in tins, but if you have to use canned clams for a cocktail dip or eat canned tuna, sardines, or salmon once in a while, perhaps it won't make a great difference.

Commercially canned fruit is packed in syrup made of sugar. Some companies now market fruit in unsweetened juice. They're still quite sweet and, accordingly, high in fructose, which feeds

Candida, so use them sparingly or not at all. Remember to boil them for ten minutes if you're especially mold-sensitive.

Approach leftovers with caution because mold forms rather quickly. If leftovers can be cooked, you should heat them at high temperature for ten minutes. The best thing to do with leftover food is to let it cool and freeze it shortly after the meal if you're planning on using it several days later. Freezing is also advisable with regard to any other uneaten foodstuffs, like crackers, quickbreads, homemade muffins, and leftover soups. At any given time, my freezer is likely to be stocked with yeast-free bread, brown rice wafers, chicken legs, frozen vegetables, sauces I've made for pastas, nuts, chips, cooked cocktail meatballs, and a stick of butter. Freezing food you're not using at the moment is not only a healthy habit, it teaches you to economize.

Avoid Chemicals, Additives, and Preservatives

Since many people with Candida react strongly to chemicals and additives, and since you're better off without most of them anyway, it's best to avoid them. There's a multitude of chemicals added to food and listed on the outside of the package or can, which should be avoided. Certain common artificial food colorings such as red dye no. 3 and yellow dye no. 5 are usually unnecessarily added to food and should be avoided. Not only are many adults allergic to them, they can cause thyroid tumors and chromosomal damage. They're also a common cause of hyperactivity in children. Acquiring knowledge about chemical additives is essential and therefore covered in greater detail later.

Eliminate Peanuts and Pistachios

Pistachios lend themselves to developing mold, and peanuts often contain a naturally-occurring toxin called "aflatoxin," so you should select walnuts, almonds, hazelnuts, pecans, and pine nuts instead. Since they tend to dry out and acquire mold, find a shop that carries very fresh, raw, unprocessed nuts; and buy them in bulk. Eat them raw or toast them as follows: Preheat the oven to 350°, spread the nuts in a pan or on a sheet of foil, and put them in the oven for ten minutes or less, checking them frequently to avoid burning; you don't want to dry out the oils in them. Remember that anything smoked or burnt doesn't serve your purposes. Always cool them thoroughly before packaging to avoid forming moisture. Store them in the fridge in a glass jar, or in the freezer in plastic bags. Leaving them in containers or plastic bags unrefrigerated for any length of time can allow mold formation and loss of nutrients and flavor.

Maintain a Hygienic Kitchen and Refrigerator

Also worth mentioning is the importance of maintaining a very clean kitchen and refrigerator. If you're going to extremes to avoid mold and contaminants, there would be no point in letting rotten food or grime accumulate on the burners, the sides of the stove, the broiler, the butcher block table, the baking board, or any location where moisture is likely to collect. Try not to leave food particles or food stains on the doorknobs of your kitchen cabinets, allowing mold to form there. Don't let dirty dishes sit around too long, and treat yourself to a clean dish towel *very frequently.*

You can use Chlorox®, Zephiran (found in drugstores), borax, white vinegar, or other mold killers when you clean. Let the refrigerator air out frequently, and see that it's cleaned on a regular basis; letting unused food or leftovers rot in the fridge generates mold and makes more problems for you later. Remember that breathing mold can aggravate your symptoms!

If you want to have an idea of how mold-ridden your home really is, mold cultures and colony counts can be taken in the kitchen and other rooms of your home. Mold plates ($15.00 each) and related information can be obtained by writing to: Sherry A. Rogers, M.D., 2800 West Genesee Street, Syracuse, New York, 13219.

CHAPTER FIVE

The Rotating Diet

If you find that you have food allergies, you should examine your eating patterns. An allergy-prone person who eats the same foods over and over can quite easily develop new allergies. In 1934, Dr. Herbert Rinkel developed a method of rotating foods which he called "The Rotary Diversified Diet"; it involves eating all regularly consumed foods on a four-day rotating schedule. This means that if you eat chicken and carrots on Monday, you shouldn't include them in your diet again before Friday. The idea of four days was adopted because it takes three days for the body to eliminate food, and a four-day policy is considered safer than three.

The rotating aspect of the regimen for candidiasis is not necessary for everybody; however, it can prove very helpful to the large number of Candida dieters who have food allergies. The rotating schedule is thus incorporated into this book and is highly recommended for people who have multiple food allergies. Rotating is one of the more challenging aspects of the Candida regimen (it even beats breakfast), and without a doubt, the one requiring the most thought, advanced planning, and discipline.

The four-day plan for rotating foods was a great discovery for more than one reason. It not only can help keep you from developing allergies to foods included in your regular regimen, it can provide a way of identifying previously unrecognized allergens. If a given food is not already in your system at the time it's eaten on the four-day plan, it's easier to detect the initial signs of an allergic reaction.

Principles of the Rotating Diet

Increase the variety of foods in your diet. At this point in time, when produce markets and grocery chains offer an extraordinary selection of foods from land, sea, and animal farms, it's amazing that most people continue to eat chicken, beef, potatoes, eggs, wheat, milk, cheese, and sugar over and over. Diversity is vital, both for nutritional considerations and, in the case of the rotating program, to minimize the risk of developing new allergies.

Eat foods in a simple, unadulterated form. Eating a lamb stew which might contain eight or nine different ingredients (including seasonings) will make it very difficult to unmask what it is you're sensitive to, if a reaction occurs. Instead of making a meat loaf with various stretchers and seasonings at home, why not make a ground beef patty, especially in the beginning when trying to track down your allergens. The principle of making simple choices is especially important when eating in a restaurant, because you won't have complete knowledge of the ingredients used.

Rotate your foods and rotate the food families. The logic here is to have the body get over the effects of a given food before having it again. If you have shrimp on Wednesday, you shouldn't have it again until Sunday. If you're inclined to eat fish shortly after the shrimp, wait until two days later; have the shrimp on Wednesday and the fish on Friday because they both come from the sea. If beef or veal (they're the same animal) is eaten on Tuesday, you shouldn't have either of them again before Saturday; and on the day after you eat beef, you shouldn't eat lamb, because they're relatives. Tomatoes, members of the nightshade family, are relatives of peppers, eggplant, and potatoes, which are also nightshades, and shouldn't be eaten one after the other. (I should add that the nightshade vegetables should be of special interest to people with arthritis, because it's possible to have an inflammatory reaction from substances called "solanines" and "solacins" found in vegetables of this family.) It's worth familiarizing yourself with some of the essential food families listed at the end of this chapter.

It's important to be aware that when you're eating apple sauce, apple juice, or apple muffins, they're all counted as *apple* when you're rotating foods. Harder to zero in on might be the wheat in the matzo meal "breading" on your veal cutlet, or the wheat in pasta and most pancakes. Be on guard because wheat is pervasive.

Avoid all foods to which you are allergic. It's easier to track down unknown allergens when reactions produced by already identified allergens are not in progress. If new foods you experiment with produce no reaction, you can add them to your diet.

As mentioned before, not all allergies are fixed. Allergies you weren't born with can often be dropped by eliminating an allergenic food from your diet for anywhere from two to six months. This is well worth pursuing because it might allow you to reintroduce certain foods into your daily regimen.

If you're a universal reactor, one who reacts allergically to most foods, eat only the foods to which you have lesser reactions to avoid starvation. You should also make every effort to locate a health care provider qualified in immunology for help in dealing with the situation, which, left to your own devices, could be extremely difficult.

The following chart provides basic guidelines for a rotating plan. It should be tailored to meet your own needs.

Eight Day Rotating Plan of Principal Food Choices

	Day 1	Day 2	Day 3	Day 4	Day 5	Day 6	Day 7	Day 8
Breakfast	Eggs	Tofu	Rice	Buck-wheat	Oats	Tofu	Rye	Lentils
Lunch	Chicken	Lentils	Salad	Pork	Eggs	Chick peas	Salad	Turkey
Dinner	Veal	Fish	Turkey	Shell-fish	Chicken	Fish	Lamb	Shell-fish

The best way to guarantee success with the four-day rotating schedule is to plan ahead and stock both freezer and refrigerator. This should be emphasized, because if you keep coming home and finding only meat loaf in the refrigerator, you'll be eating beef all the time or skipping meals altogether. If you do well with fruit, you should have four different fruits in the fridge at all times for rotating purposes. But try to avoid letting rot and mold form on them. It's also good thinking to have four different frozen vegetables on hand, provided they don't contain chemicals. For late-night snacks, you should have on hand, also in varieties of four, the "munchies" mentioned in Chapter Nine (The Emergency Survival Kit). Going to bed with nagging hunger can promote sleeplessness.

If you choose to have herb tea for breakfast, this too should be taken on a rotating basis. The ingredients on the boxes should be carefully scrutinized for existing or potential allergens. Buying a number of teas that contain the same ingredients isn't recommended. For example, many herb teas contain rose hips, hibiscus flowers, camomile and other herbs in varying combinations. If you continue to have these same ingredients in different teas day after day, you can develop sensitivities to them. Here's a plan which should minimize the risk of developing sensitivities to herb teas.

> Day One: Cranberry Cove by Celestial Seasonings
> Day Two: Camomile Flowers by Pompadour
> Day Three: Huckleberry Leaf by Lion
> Day Four: Verveine by Pompadour.

The next time Day One comes around, you can begin to repeat the process with Cranberry Cove, or choose another tea which also contains cinnamon and rosehips. An herb tea such as Emperor's Choice by Celestial Seasonings isn't recommended because it contains eleven different ingredients; if you react to the tea, it will be hard to identify what's causing the reaction. You can also make your own tea by boiling fresh herbs, such as mint or fennel; or try boiling cherry stems like the French.

How far should you go with rotation? You don't have to become a fanatic about the four-day scheme, but the more religious, the more results. I know some people who go so far as to use four different sugar-free, chemical-free toothpastes.

Seven-Day Menu Plan Incorporating the Four-Day Rotation Diet

Day One
Breakfast: Onion omelet; steamed carrots; herb tea
Lunch: Broiled salmon with tossed salad—*or*—canned water-pack salmon on lettuce with avocado, carrots, red onions, and lemon mayonnaise
Dinner: Broiled scallops; baked potato with butter or oil *or* petite peas *or* corn; escarole *or* kale *or* cauliflower *or* cabbage (red or white)

Day Two
Breakfast: Rice cake with almond, sunflower, or sesame butter; herb tea (different from Day One)
Lunch: Sautéed chicken, bell peppers, and zucchini with toasted almonds *or* hazelnuts *or* pecans, garlic, and

ginger (seasonings optional); small portion of rice

Dinner: Roast chicken with rolled oats (or barley flakes) dressing; Brussels sprouts *or* zucchini; white turnips *or* rutabagas

Day Three

Breakfast: Tofu cocktail *or* fresh pear (if fruit allowed); veal patty; string beans *or* wax beans (butter beans); herb tea (different from Day One and Day Two)

Lunch: Stir-fried shrimp with snow peas, string beans, and pine nuts *or* water chestnuts (or both)

Dinner: Broiled veal chop; patty pan *or* yellow summer squash; beets *or* lima beans *or* parsnips *or* butternut squash

Day Four

Breakfast: Buckwheat pancakes *or* waffles with unsweetened apple sauce; herb tea (different from Day One, Day Two, and Day Three)

Lunch: Salade Niçoise: canned water-pack tuna *or* sardines *or* crab meat tossed with lettuce, cucumbers, tomatoes, radishes, scallions, and black olives (optional); dressing of lime juice, olive oil, and fresh basil

Dinner: Broiled halibut *or* swordfish *or* other fish; steamed fresh asparagus *or* frozen artichoke hearts; tomato broiled with oil, thyme, onion powder, salt, and pepper

Day Five

Breakfast: Lentil soup with carrots, celery, shallots, and herbs; herb tea (Day One choice can be repeated here)

Lunch: Spinach and goat cheese omelet with side of petite green peas and shallots; green salad with fresh orange juice, vegetable oil, and fresh herbs of your choice; two rye crackers

Dinner: Broiled lamb chops; spinach *or* kale; steamed cauliflower *or* broiled eggplant

Day Six

Breakfast: Two small rice muffins sweetened with banana *or* canned sugar-free pineapple *or* fresh peach—*or*—corn bread (if not allergic to corn); herb tea (Day Two choice can be repeated here)

Lunch: Stir-fried chicken, broccoli, onions, and zucchini *or* red bell peppers with garlic and ginger (seasonings optional); small portion of rice (preferably brown)—*or*—homemade chicken soup with vegetables and rice

Dinner: Roast turkey *or* duck; parsnips *or* rutabagas; zucchini *or* Brussels sprouts *or* broccoli

Day Seven

Breakfast: Oatmeal; nuts of your choice; herb tea (Day Three choice can be repeated here)

Lunch: Beef or veal patty, well drained; potatoes (mashed or steamed) *or* parsnips; green salad with lemon and oil dressing *or* homemade coleslaw *or* string beans vinaigrette (lemon juice and oil)

Dinner: Broiled shrimp with lemon butter and parsley; patty pan *or* yellow summer squash *or* wax beans (butter beans); cooked cabbage *or* escarole *or* okra

Cheating on the Diet

Since almost everybody seems to weaken and binge on the diet or on the forbidden allergens once in a while, it's important to note that such a mishap can be remedied, if it doesn't happen too often. You can contact your health professional and follow his or her advice to get yourself back on track. Sometimes this involves returning to an earlier stage of treatment and using "first phase" strategies, such as antioxidants and bulking substances (i.e. dietary fiber such as oat bran, psyllium husks, guar gum, or glucomannon).

Two procedures I recommend strongly are to drink a great deal of water and to encourage as complete a bowel movement as possible, to detoxify yourself. These are good habits to adopt on a regular basis anyway, because the more cleansed the intestinal tract, the better you'll feel.

I should also mention that on those few and far between occasions when I'm at a dinner party and I find myself indulging, I take an additional amount of my anti-yeast medication *while I'm having the forbidden foods and beverages* as a way of counteracting the potential for Candida growth. While I'm not recommending that you cheat, it's important to know what steps to take if the need arises.

FOOD FAMILIES

PLANT FAMILIES

AGAR
mushroom
yeast

APPLE
apple
    apple cider
    apple vinegar
pear
quince

BANANA
banana
plantain

BEECH
beechnuts
chestnuts

BIRCH
filbert
hazelnut

BUCKWHEAT
buckwheat
rhubarb
sorrel

CASHEW
cashew
mango
pistachio

CITRUS
citron
grapefruit

kumquat
lemon
lime
orange
tangerine

COMPOSITE
absinthe
camomile
chicory
artichoke
dandelion
endive
escarole
Jerusalem artichoke
lettuce
oyster plant
safflower
salsify
sunflower

CYPERACEAE
Chinese water chestnut

GINGER
cardamom
ginger
turmeric

GINSENG
ginseng

GOOSEBERRY
currant
gooseberry

GOOSEFOOT
beet
   beet sugar
spinach
Swiss chard

GOURD
cucumber
   gherkin
muskmelon
   cantaloupe
   casaba
   honeydew
   Persian melon
   Spanish melon
pumpkin
summer squash
watermelon
winter squash

GRAINS (GRASSES)
bamboo
barley
corn
   grits
   meal
   starch
   sugar (syrup)
      dextrose
      glucose
millet
oats
rice
rye
sorghum
sugar cane
   molasses
wheat
   bran
   farina
   flour

gluten
graham
germ
semolina
triticale
wild rice

GRAPE
grape
   brandy
   champagne
   cream of tartar
   raisin
   vinegar
   wine

HEATHER
blueberry
cranberry
huckleberry

IRIS
saffron

LAUREL
avocado
cinnamon
sassafras

LECYTHIS
Brazil nut

LEGUMES
black-eyed pea
carob
chickpea (garbanzo)
garbanzo bean (chickpea)
kidney bean
lentil
licorice
lima bean

mung bean
navy bean
pea
peanut
pinto bean
soybean
 lecithin
 tofu
string bean

LILY
aloe
asparagus
chives
garlic
leek
onion
yucca

MACADAMIA
macadamia nuts

MADDER
coffee

MALLOW
cottonseed
okra

MAPLE
maple sugar
maple syrup

MINT
basil
catnip
lavender
marjoram
mint
oregano
peppermint

rosemary
sage
savory
spearmint
thyme

MORNING GLORY
sweet potato
yam

MULBERRY
breadfruit
fig
mulberry

MUSTARD
broccoli
Brussels sprouts
cabbage
cauliflower
collards
kale
kohlrabi
mustard
rutabaga
turnip

MYRTLE
allspice
clove
guava
paprika
pimento

NUTMEG
mace
nutmeg

OLIVE
olive

ORCHID
vanilla

PALM
coconut
date palm
dates
sago

PAPAYA
anise
caraway
carrot
celery
dill
fennel
parsley
parsnip

PEPPER
black pepper
white pepper

PINE
juniper
pine nut

PINEAPPLE
pineapple

PLUM
almond
apricot
cherry
nectarine
peach
plum

prune

POMEGRANATE
pomegranate

POPPY
poppy seed

NIGHTSHADE
chili
eggplant
pepper
    capsicum
    cayenne
potato
tobacco
tomato

PURSLANE
New Zealand spinach
purslane

ROSE
blackberry
boysenberry
raspberry
strawberry

STERCULA
cocoa
    chocolate
cola

TEA
tea

ANIMAL FAMILIES

AMPHIBIANS
frog

BIRDS
chicken
duck
goose
grouse
pheasant
quail
guinea fowl
turkey
pigeon

CRUSTACEANS
shrimp
lobster
crab
crayfish

FISH
shark
sturgeon
    caviar
tarpon
herring
shad
anchovy
sardine
salmon
    caviar
trout
whitefish
smelt
pike
pickerel
buffalo
carp

catfish
eel
scrod
cod
haddock
pollack
hake
mullet
barracuda
bass
    rockfish
grouper
perch
snapper
    tile
black bass
sunfish
bluefish
pompano
amberjack
mackerel (jack)
mackerel
    Atlantic
    Spanish
    king
    frigate
croaker
weakfish
whiting
drumfish
porgy
tuna
swordfish
butterfish
flounder
halibut
sole

INSECTA
honeybee

MAMMALS
rabbit
squirrel
beaver
whale
dolphin
bear
raccoon
elephant
horse
pig
llama
deer
elk
moose
reindeer

cattle
buffalo
sheep (lamb)
goat

MOLLUSKS
scallop
oyster
quahog
clam
abalone
snail
squid
octopus

REPTILES
turtle
rattlesnake
alligator

CHAPTER SIX

Shopping and Reading Labels: Is It "Candida Kosher"?

Unless you're a person of unlimited leisure, you'll probably want to confine your heavy-duty shopping trips to two or so per week. If you shop even more frequently than that, you'll probably be eating fresher produce, which is of supreme importance on this diet. You should buy fresh meat, fish, and fowl whenever possible, but if you're not going to consume these foods right away, by all means freeze them. There are some foodstuffs on the diet, like cereals, rice, dried beans, snacks and chips, oils, butter, and nut butters, that can be bought either in volume or as they run out.

Some people have a natural talent for detective work and lend themselves to uncovering clues and digging for buried information. People who have Candida and who lack this skill should try to acquire it, not only to help identify trouble-making allergies, but to examine labels in food stores. In the early days of dieting, you may find yourself buying a number of products, only to discover when you get home that you can't eat them because they're not "Candida kosher," that is, not pure as defined by the guidelines of the Candida diet. In order to avoid a costly pitfall, why not carry this book to the market until you're totally familiar with what's allowed and not allowed on the diet. If you wear glasses for reading, don't leave them at home when you shop, because careful scrutiny of every label is in order.

Avoiding the No-Nos

In choosing products, you should read *everything* on the front of the can or package, as well as the list of ingredients, which can be found almost anywhere on the label. Bear in mind that the contents of a product are listed in order of weight. Thus, if a label reads "Tomatoes, onions, peppers, garlic powder, and salt," you know there are more tomatoes than onions and more garlic powder than salt.

At the risk of being repetitious, let me reiterate that it's important to avoid any product containing an ingredient to which you're allergic. This requires knowing what your allergies are, and the sooner you find out, the better. If you're in the dark about this, like so many people who have allergies, consult the chapter called "Allergy" for assistance in this complex matter.

Other substances to identify and avoid are soy sauce, tamari, vinegar, cheese, sour cream, buttermilk, kefir, MSG, yeast, and malt. You should also be on the lookout for such prominent no-nos as peanuts, pistachios, dried fruits, smoked foods, alcohol, and foods containing alcohol, like vanilla extract, plus the full range of sweeteners, which includes dextrose, honey, molasses, date sugar, maple sugar, turbinado sugar, corn and maple syrups, sorbitol, Equal® (NutraSweet®), saccharin, and any other chemical sweeteners. As mentioned before, staying away from canned foods, to the extent possible, is also recommended.

When reading labels, be sure to consider the carbohydrate gram count, if it's given. For example, on the back of a bag of El Molino Puffed Rice Cereal, it says that the serving size is ¾ of a cup and the carbohydrate gram count for that amount is twelve. One knows it's possible to work twelve grams into the daily carbohydrate count. However, if the count for an item is 48 grams per serving, be aware that it's a high count for one serving.

Another consideration in shopping involves what your doctor may have indicated as applicable to *you*. Looking at the sodium and/or cholesterol content in products (if noted) may be important in *your* case. Or remembering that eating too much meat can affect your kidneys or raise your uric acid to an abnormal level might apply to you. In any case, it's the patient who should take prime responsibility for monitoring these factors.

You'll find many surprises at the supermarket. Pasta, for example, is thought to be free of yeast; yet, on a recent shopping trip, I noticed that Buitoni pasta products, unlike others in my supermarket, contain dried yeast. Some bottled or canned spaghetti sauces contain sugar, corn syrup, or corn sweeteners; such sauces may also contain fermented cheese and/or dextrose, all of which are not allowed on the Candida diet. Fortunately, there are some bottled pasta sauces, like Enrico's and DeBoles Marinara (found at the health food store), which are Candida kosher. On my shopping trip, I also looked at two canned clam sauces out of curiosity; one contained dextrose and the other cornstarch, which would be a problem for people allergic to corn. Picking up some Streit's whole wheat matzo crackers, I discovered that they're free of both yeast and malt; not *all* matzo crackers are malt-free. Some companies list ingredients in a way that's tricky. P & Q Tomato Ketchup (an A&P product) lists "natural sweeteners" as an ingredient; how do we know they don't consider sugar a natural sweetener? When in doubt, it's best to leave the product on the shelf.

Another category of ingredients to steer clear of are the chemicals and preservatives contained in commercially-marketed products. Several thousand different compounds (literally) are added to packaged foods in order to save the consumer's time, improve color and flavor, prolong shelf life, and increase corporate profits. If you're sensitive to chemicals, as many Candida patients are, you may have an allergic reaction to some of the foods that contain them. But apart from that, a whole host of chemicals commonly added to foods are not yet known to be safe. The U.S. Federal Drug Administration (USFDA) has what's called the Generally Recognized As Safe (GRAS) list, which, in fact, contains many chemicals that have never been tested for safety but which are used by food manufacturers. According to Beatrice Trum Hunter in her very informative work, *Additives Book*, an FDA official even went so far as to state publicly that the agency is not bound to remove a substance from the GRAS list on the basis of initial, but isolated, evidence of potential danger that isn't widely accepted by scientists. "GRAS doesn't have to mean unanimously recognized as safe," he added.

You should become familiar with some of the chemicals and other food additives contained in commercial products; it's wise to know what you're buying and become educated as to the hazardous nature of some of these substances. You can't expect profit-minded industry to enlighten you. See the list of chemicals and additives commonly used in American food products included in this chapter.

Pesticides, hormones, residues of substances used to process food, and antibiotics (the use of which can cause Candida in the first place) can all be found, potentially, in the food we buy.

Hormones are used to make cows grow faster and develop more plumpness in order to yield a better financial gain. Antibiotics keep food from spoiling while it's being stored, transported, or prepared for freezing. They're also used to stave off disease in fish, poultry, and meat-producing animals. The ice on which fish is displayed is sometimes treated with antibiotics. This is a good reason to wash fish well before cooking. There isn't a great deal you can do to counteract the antibiotics used in and on food except to treat your yeast problem with the hope of making yourself less vulnerable. The use of antibiotics in the food supply is said to be under review by the FDA.

The Great Letter Writing Campaign

Think of all the people who will probably develop Candida in the future because of the continued and widespread use of antibiotics, birth control pills, and steroids, among other factors. It won't be any easier for them, since the use of food additives shows little sign of abating, and air and water pollution around the world are unquestionably on the rise. None of this will change unless you and your children, the young people who'll be living during the very advanced stages of pollution, take the situation in hand and put pressure on the powers that be. Two of the main sources of pollution in New York are the city's buses and the federal government's mail trucks. Yes, the government is one of the primary offenders! The private sanitation trucks entering the city each day to collect refuse from various commercial enterprises are outrageous generators of poisonous fumes and summonses from the Air Resources Bureau are few and far between. This isn't a book about pollution in New York City or the negligence of public officials, but the subject is very relevant in that the more pollution you're exposed to, the harder it is to treat and get your candidiasis under control. Speak to your sons and daughters who haven't had their cars tuned up. Write to your president, governor, mayor, the chairman of the Environmental Protection Agency in Washington, your congresspeople, your U.S. and state senators, and the local environmental protection organization which isn't giving out the necessary summonses. The sooner you do this, the sooner the problem will be addressed on the large scale that's needed.

As for making life easier for people with Candida in relation to food, you can write the U.S. Department of Agriculture, the U.S. Food and Drug Administration, and your congresspeople, asking them to demand that all food additives on the GRAS list be tested for safety. You should also write to the companies who make crackers, snacks, cereals, and frozen muffins, asking them to make products free of yeast, sugar, vinegar, soy sauce, tamari, malt, and unnecessary preservatives. There are many products free of sugar on the market now, but in too many cases, honey or chemical sweeteners have taken the place of sugar. It's important for manufacturers to understand that foods like crackers and cereals don't need sweeteners at all, and if properly packaged, many of them don't need preservatives either.

Then you should write the companies who *do* make yeast-free, sugar-free, chemical-free products, expressing your appreciation for their contribution to the field of nutrition and health and encourage them to develop more products free of these ingredients. It'll only happen if there's demand from the consumer. That's how low-sodium products came to exist in the marketplace.

You'd also be providing a great service if you wrote the national supermarket chains and the important smaller chains in your area, asking them to carry more health food products such as cold-pressed oils, sugar-free and yeast-free foods, chemical-free potato chips, cereals free of malt and sugar, and other foods you buy on a regular basis. You may want to attach a list of specific products, giving the names of the companies that market them. See the list of food products containing some of this information at the end of this chapter. If supermarkets carried more of the products now found exclusively in health food stores, not only would the products be more accessible to the public, the prices on these items would probably be reduced because their mass manufacture would enable producers to sell them for less.

Unfortunately, the world isn't heavily populated with people like Ralph Nader, David Horowitz, and Betty Furness. These good souls have accomplished wonders, but they need an army of people behind them. You and I have to be the majors and lieutenants in that army, and writing is one of the ways this particular army will gain ground. In writing letters to elected officials, government agencies, and manufacturers, you can have a greater impact on them by composing additional letters from your family members and friends (with their permission) and having them sign their own names. You can also have additional people add their signatures to letters written under your name. Everyone isn't willing to take the time, and many people aren't naturals for letter-writing.

Another way you can effect change is by using your dollar to register a protest. If you want cattle farmers to drop the use of antibiotics and hormones on cows, and if you want the beef industry to process only animals free of illness for meat, stop buying beef! If you want California farmers to stop using herbicides on the soil, pesticides on plants and trees, and wax and sprayed coatings on produce, boycott California produce. They'll find a new technology! As we saw with the use of alar on fruit crops, the public can make a lot of noise in the media, but holding back the dollar gets speedy results!

Chemicals and Other Additives Commonly Used in Commercially-Marketed Foods

The following list is intended to provide useful information on some of the chemicals and additives commonly used in commercially-marketed foods. Remember that this information changes constantly because there's a great deal of controversy surrounding some of the chemicals and additives used in our American food supply. There are also new discoveries and new rulings all the time. If you'd like additional information on chemicals and additives, look for a recently published book on the subject at the health food store.

Ascorbic acid—An inexpensive, safe additive used as a vitamin supplement (vitamin C) in beverages, potato flakes, and breakfast foods. Ascorbic acid functions both as an oxidant to promote the oxidation of food and an antioxidant to prevent the oxidation of food. It's used by bakers to make bread knead more easily and to give the loaf a finer texture, but doesn't provide anything nutritional when used in bread because it's destroyed in the baking process. Some people take as much as 6,000 milligrams or more of ascorbic acid each day in powdered or tablet form to bolster the immune system.

Aspartame—A sugar substitute discovered in 1965. It's made from two amino acids and processed in the body as a natural food. Marketed as NutraSweet® and Equal®, it's used to replace saccharin in diet beverages. In 1970, aspartic acid, a component of aspartame, was found to produce lesions in test mice. In 1983, there were reports on aspartame that revealed side effects in humans. Aspartame can provoke reactions in individuals sensitive to milk because it's cut with milk sugar.

Artificial food colors—Coal tar dyes used to make food more visually appealing. Without them, frankfurters would be gray, fruit sodas would be colorless, frozen sherbet would be pale, and manufacturers would probably make less money. The following colors are still in use: Blue nos. 1 and 2; green no.3; red nos. 3 and 40; yellow nos. 5 and 6. Much controversy surrounds the use of artificial food colors. Red no. 3 has shown adverse effects on blood. It was also found to be carcinogenic in the early 1980's. Some individuals are allergic to yellow no. 5 (tartrazine); this is often true of people sensitive to aspirin. Thanks to Dr. Ben Feingold, we now know that artificial colorings are one of the causes of hyperactivity in children. Some manufacturers are beginning to turn to natural sources of coloring, such as saffron, paprika, carrot oil, annatto, and dehydrated beets.

Benzoic acid—A preservative found in some fruit juices and fruit preserves, in bottled soft drinks, and in pickles. Benzoic acid is sometimes added as a flavoring in ices, ice cream, chewing gum, candy, and baked goods, and to retard mold in harvested crops and in food packaging materials. It's used in small amounts (0.05% or 0.10%) in foods and is classified by the government as "generally recognized as safe."

Beta-carotene—An important nutritional supplement which the body converts to vitamin A as needed. It's found in green leafy vegetables, yellow fruits and vegetables, and egg yolk. Synthetic beta-carotene is added to milk, butter, margarine, non-dairy creamers, and cake mixes as a means of coloring; it also adds nutrition. Beta-carotene is advertised by companies who make nutritional supplements as effective in protecting humans from cancer. If taken in unusually large doses, the storage of carotene in the body can give the skin an orange pigmentation, which fades away slowly when the substance is eliminated from the diet. It's considered non-toxic.

BHA (butylated hydroxyanisole) and BHT (butylated hydroxytoluene)—Prevent polyunsaturated oils from oxidizing, extend shelf life, and keep food from becoming rancid. Usually listed on packages, they're very often found in food containing fats or oil and breakfast cereals, spices, snacks, and processed meats. Their use is often unnecessary. BHA and BHT can cause hyperactivity in children and allergic reactions in some individuals. They can also affect reproduction adversely. In 1986, BHA was found to be a carcinogen and BHT a probable carcinogen. The research continues, while safer alternatives like vitamins C and E begin to replace them.

Caffeine—A stimulant which acts on the central nervous system. Nature lends caffeine to tea leaves, coffee, cocoa, and kola beans. It's used as an additive in chocolate and soft drinks. Consumption of too much caffeine can produce symptoms such as irregular heartbeat, headaches, and anxiety. The tolerance level for caffeine varies greatly. It's been proven to cause birth defects in animals, and is considered hazardous to pregnant women (especially in the first three months) and nursing mothers. Some individuals are allergic to caffeine; anyone with a gastrointestinal or cardiovascular problem should also stay away from it. There's much more research to be done on caffeine.

Calcium disodium EDTA—A substance that ties up and deactivates metal ions (a sequestrant) in food to keep it from discoloring or turning rancid. EDTA is used to retain color and enhance the flavor of vinegar, pickled cucumbers, canned carbonated soft drinks, certain canned cooked vegetables, canned seafoods, and products containing hard boiled eggs. Since it prevents oil from turning rancid, it's also used as a preservative in mayonnaise, some sauces, salad dressings, sandwich spreads, and margarines. If consumed at normal levels, calcium disodium EDTA is considered safe.

Calcium propionate and sodium propionate—Ingredients occurring naturally in dairy products. Calcium propionate is commonly used to inhibit the growth of fungi and some bacteria in baked bread products, processed cheeses, and chocolate products, among other foods. Sodium propionate is mostly found in cakes, pies, and other pastries. When used, these chemicals reduce the losses for bakers because fewer baked products are returned as stale. While not considered harmful, they're known to induce allergic reactions and migraines in some individuals.

Carrageenan—Seaweed, also known as Irish Moss. It's used as a gelling agent in puddings, a suspending agent in chocolate milk drinks, and a stabilizer in fruit juices and soft drinks. It's also used to clarify wine and beer, to control beer foam, to prevent oil and water from separating, and to make cream cheese more spreadable. Toothpastes, deodorants, and hand lotions often contain carrageenan. Since it has produced dead fetuses and some birth defects in rats and mice, it should be avoided by pregnant women until further study is completed. Carrageenan was removed from the GRAS list in 1972.

Casein—The principal protein in milk. Casein is used as a thickener and whitener. It's found in frozen custard, ice cream, sherbet, and non-dairy creamers. While considered nutritious, it should be avoided by individuals allergic to cow's milk.

Citric acid (sodium citrate)—A naturally occurring substance in pineapple, apricots, some berries, citrus fruits, and tomatoes. It's widely used in commercial products such as canned seafood, canned tomatoes, and bottled roasted peppers. Manufacturers make it from the fermentative action of *Aspergillus niger,* a fungus found in sugar beet molasses. It's economical and serves as an antioxidant in products such as instant mashed potatoes and potato sticks; it's also used to trap metal ions in wine. Citric acid is found in some over-the-counter medications. It's considered safe.

Corn syrup—A thick, sweet solution made from corn. It's used to thicken and sweeten certain foods and drinks; when dried and used in powdered products, it's called "corn syrup solids." Corn syrup contains dextrin, dextrose, and maltose. Although safe, it should be avoided by diabetics and Candida patients.

Daminozide (alar)—A chemical used on crops such as apples and cherries for uniform ripening. There's much consumer awareness of and action against the use of alar. The Environmental Protection Agency found it to be a carcinogen in 1984 and finally lowered the permissible levels of use in 1987. Due to consumer protest, many supermarkets refuse to sell fruit treated with alar.

Dextrose (glucose)—A chemical present in all living cells. When we eat starch, the digestive enzymes in our bodies break it down to dextrose (sugar), which is used for energy. The body also converts dextrose to glycogen, which is stored and then converted back to dextrose when we need energy. It's used by manufacturers as a sweetener; it also lends body to soft drinks and gives caramels their brown color. It's about 25 percent less sweet than cane sugar. Dextrose nourishes Candida.

Ferrous gluconate—An iron salt present in the human body. Ferrous gluconate is widely used for darkening olives, which can vary in color tone. This process is considered safe.

Guar gum—A popular and inexpensive vegetable gum stabilizer from the guar gum plant. The seeds from the guar gum plant, which resembles the soybean plant, provide a valuable source of protein for livestock. Guar gum serves as a thickening agent in salad dressings, frozen puddings, drinks, and ice cream. It's also used to make dough and batter more resilient. Though not viewed as a hazard to health, its safety for pregnant women has not been determined.

Hydrolyzed vegetable protein or HVP—Usually derived from soybeans and composed of amino acids. HVP is used in gravies, sauces, soups, stews, frankfurters, and canned chili to enhance the natural flavor of food. It's considered safe.

Lactic acid/calcium lactate—Found in every living organism. Lactic acid is used by the food industry to keep green olives from spoiling, to add tartness to soda drinks and frozen desserts, and to regulate acidity in the cheese-making process. It's excreted in the body's urine. Calcium lactate is the non-acidic salt of lactic acid; it prevents processed fruits and vegetables from changing color and improves the quality of baked goods and condensed and powdered milk. Lactic acid is considered safe at levels used in food, but could cause problems when added to the formulas of infants under three months of age.

Lecithin—A very inexpensive waste product of the soybean industry. Lecithin can also come from egg yolks, but at a much higher cost. While it's used as an antioxidant in oils, margarine, and shortening to prevent rancidity, its principal use is as an emulsifier (to help fat or oil mix with water) in baked goods, chocolate, margarine, and ice cream. In margarine, lecithin prevents water leakage, protects the beta-carotene, and reduces the spattering effect when used in frying. Lecithin found in egg yolk serves as a natural emulsifier in foods like mayonnaise. Many individuals take commercially-marketed soya lecithin capsules to supplement their diets. Some health professionals say it helps lower cholesterol levels in the system. It's considered non-toxic and nutritious.

Mannitol—A sugar alcohol used as a sweetener in sugarless chewing gum and as a powdered coating on ordinary gum to prevent gum from absorbing moisture. Mannitol is used in low-calorie foods because it generates only half the calories of ordinary sugar. It can serve as a diuretic for medical use and can have a laxative effect if used in doses higher than what's normally used in food products. While considered safe, it's not recommended for Candida patients because the body converts it to sugar.

Methylene chloride—A chemical solvent that, in the 1970's, replaced trichloroethylene in the process of extracting caffeine from coffee. Methylene chloride is also used as a propellant or solvent in cosmetics. Since it was found to cause cancer in test animals, some coffee producers have switched to other substances for removing caffeine, but no labeling of the method is required.

Modified food starches—Used as coaters, fillers, binders, and diluters, as well as anti-sticking, bulking and absorbing agents. Modified food starches are used to give a smooth texture to pie fillings, and sheen and stability to baked goods; they also stabilize commercial frostings and cream fillings. They're added to baby foods to replace more nutritious, costly ingredients, and to make these foods appear more substantial and more appetizing. Canned foods like sauces, gravies, chili, soups, and stews often contain modified starches. They're also added to baking powder and confectioners sugar to absorb moisture and prevent caking. These starches come from corn primarily, but also from wheat, sorghum, tapioca, arrowroot, and potatoes. They provide added calories and little nutrition. The safety of modified food starches won't be determined until further long-term studies are conducted.

Mono- and diglycerides—Comprise about one percent of normal food fat and are part of normal diet. Mono- and diglycerides are absorbed into the cells of the intestine and converted into triglycerides which pass into the bloodstream. Commercially they're used to make cakes fluffier, keep the oil and peanuts in peanut butter from separating, and to prevent bread from turning stale by keeping the starch from crystallizing. Several derivatives of mono- and diglycerides are also found in food products. They're considered safe and wholesome.

Monosodium glutamate (MSG)—An amino acid present in all proteins and many foods. It's used to enhance the flavor of soup, seafood, sauces, meat, poultry, and cheese. While most MSG is commercially produced by the bacterial fermentation of sugar, some comes from plant proteins rich in glutamic acid. Many individuals are vulnerable to the "Chinese restaurant syndrome," a reaction produced by MSG that may occur 20 to 30 minutes after beginning a Chinese meal; it manifests itself in headaches, tightness of chest, and other symptoms. Tests conducted on baby mice revealed that *large* amounts of MSG can cause brain damage. Pregnant women, Candida patients, and those sensitive to wheat, corn, or sugar beets (MSG is derived from these) are advised to avoid MSG.

Potassium bromate—Used to improve baking properties of flour for many years. Baking converts potassium bromate to bromide, which is absorbed when the bread is digested. Bromide, which is harmless, travels in the bloodstream and is excreted in the urine. Calcium bromate is sometimes substituted for potassium bromate.

Propyl gallate—An antioxidant used to increase shelf life of foods. Sometimes added to the packaging material used on breakfast cereals and potato flakes, it's also found in vegetable oils, shortenings, baked goods, some snack foods, candies, and gum. Propyl gallate is often used together with BHT and BHA because of the synergistic effect these three food additives have in keeping oil and fat from turning rancid. Current levels of propyl gallate used in food don't appear to pose problems, but more testing is needed to determine safety.

Sodium nitrite and sodium nitrate—Used to color and flavor processed meats and as a preservative that greatly extends shelf life. When food is treated with nitrites and heated, botulinum spores are killed off, preventing botulism food poisoning. Much publicity has surrounded the use of nitrites because they can induce the formation of cancer-causing nitrosamines. Nitrites are very high on the list of toxic chemicals used in foods; they're toxic at levels only slightly higher than the levels normally found in foods on the American market. While used less than previously, nitrites are still added to maintain the freshness of salami, frankfurters, ham, bacon, and smoked fish. Nitrite-free meats are labeled accordingly. Research has revealed that nitrites can have adverse effects on infants when consumed during pregnancy.

Sorbitol—A sugar alcohol like mannitol and xylitol. Sorbitol extends shelf life because it keeps sugar from crystallizing. It's used in dietetic ice cream, candy, and chewing gum. Although sorbitol is more slowly absorbed than normal sugars like cane, corn, and beet, it's still absorbed into the bloodstream where it's converted to sugar. Manufacturers deceptively refer to it as low-calorie. Sorbitol can cause diarrhea in children and should be avoided by diabetics and people who have Candida.

Sucrose—Ordinary table sugar from sugar cane or sugar beets, as opposed to other sugars derived from sorghum, maple trees, honey, or fruit. Sucrose goes through a refining process which removes all its vitamins and protein and almost all its minerals. It's used commercially to sweeten foods and beverages. An average American is said to consume about one hundred pounds of sucrose per year. Candida loves it too.

Sulfites—Preservatives used in wines, fruits, and vegetables to mask spoilage, prevent discoloration, and discourage bacterial growth. Allergic reactions and asthmatic attacks are not uncommon after exposure to sulfites. Due to cases in which sulfites have caused deaths, the FDA has banned the use of them on most fresh fruits and vegetables. Labeling of sulfite content in dried fruit and alcoholic beverages is now required.

Vanillin—Manufactured by the chemical industry because of an insufficient supply of natural vanilla extract from the vanilla plant. Although vanillin has a similar taste, it's not considered as good as the much acclaimed natural vanilla. The body absorbs and converts vanillin to vanillic acid, and excretes both of them in the urine. Humans actually produce as much as one-half milligram of their own vanillin per day. It poses no problems when used in food products.

Xanthan gum—An additive used as a suspending agent, thickener, stabilizer, and emulsifier. It contains complex carbohydrates and is composed of sugar and sugar-acid units. Xanthan gum is produced by the controlled fermentation of dextrose and often used as a replacement for starch in foods like pie fillings and puddings. Generally speaking, this substance doesn't provoke allergic reactions and seems to pose no hazard, even when consumed in large amounts. Because of its sugar content, xanthan gum should be avoided by people on the Candida diet.

Xylitol—A sugar alcohol used as a sweetener in chewing gum and in coatings on vitamins. Used also as a sugar substitute in dietetic jams and jellies, xylitol has a laxative effect on some people and can cause flatulence and other intestinal disturbances. Mice that ingested xylitol in high doses developed bladder stones and bladder tumors; some experimental rats showed changes in the adrenal glands. Because of these findings, some manufacturers have eliminated xylitol from their products.

Sources of Candida Kosher Food Products

This list contains some commercial products (mostly found in health food stores) that are within the confines of the Candida diet (considered Candida kosher), along with the names and addresses of their manufacturers. In many cases you'll find a similar product made by a different company. That's fine, as long as you've checked the ingredients; *it's the purity of the product that matters, not the manufacturer.* Be aware that new products are developed all the time and that the ingredients in commercial products change very frequently, so certain items listed here may contain different ingredients than they did at the time I researched them. For that reason, you should read *all* ingredients carefully before buying any of the products on this list. This also applies to the other products made by these manufacturers. Please use your head: If some sugarless cereals have an abundance of raisins and dates, stay away from them unless you do especially well with dried fruits. With regard to yeast-free bread made with a culture, as in the case of sourdough, try a small amount of it and see how you do. I have yeast-free rye bread every four days, but most Candida dieters are better off with no bread at all. I sincerely hope you'll see this as a list of products to be used according to your own individual diet restrictions and the advice of your health professional.

Company	Product
After the Fall Products, Inc. Brattleboro, VT 05301	natural fruit juices
Amsnack, Inc. Stockton, CA	brown rice chips
Arrowhead Mills, Inc. Box 2059 Hereford, TX 79045	grains, whole grain flour, legumes (dried beans and lentils), corn for popping, bran, seeds, flakes of barley, rye, oat, soy, potato, wheat, Nature O's Cereal, Rice and Shine (hot cereal), Quick Brown Rice (plain version), puffed wheat, rice, corn, and millet (malt-free), muffin mixes, unrefined oils

Balanced Foods, Inc. North Bergen, NJ 07047	almond meal, pumpkin meal, sesame meal, canned low-sodium seafood, natural fruit juices, sea salt
Barbara's Bakery, Inc. Petaluma, CA 94952	cereals sweetened with fruit juice, granola sweetened with fruit juice, granola bars, potato chips
Berkshire Mountain Bakery P.O. Box 785 Housatonic, MA 01236	Richard Bourdon Sourdough Rye Bread, Richard Bourdon Sourdough Whole Wheat Bread
Birkett Mills P.O. Box 440-A Penn Yan, NY 14527	Pocono Brand roasted stone-ground buckwheat groats
The Blue Corn Connection 3825 Academy Parkway South NE Albuquerque, NM 87109	blue corn for popping
Celestial Seasonings, Inc. 1780 55th Street Boulder, CO 80301-2799	herb teas
Con Agra, Inc. Omaha, NE 68102	cream of rye
DeBoles Nutritional Foods, Inc. 2120 Jericho Turnpike Garden City Park, NY 11040	pasta, marinara, spaghetti sauce
Dimpflmeier Bakery Limited 32 Advance Road Toronto, Ontario Canada M8Z-2T4	yeast-free 100% rye bread

Eden Foods
701 Tecumseh Road
Clinton, MI 49236

legumes,
corn for popping,
unrefined oils,
unsweetened applesauce,
sea vegetable chips,
brown rice chips

Edwards & Son
Union, NJ 07083

brown rice crackers

El Molino
Division of American Health
Products, Inc.
Ramsey, NJ 07446

malt-free, sugar-free cereals

Elam Mills
2625 Gardner Road
Broadview, IL 60153-4499

unbleached flour,
bran,
steel cut oatmeal

Ener-G Foods, Inc.
6901 Fox Avenue S.
P.O. Box 84487
Seattle, WA 98124-5787

Wheat-Free Oat Baking Mix,
White Rice Baking Mix,
Yeast-Free Brown Rice Bread,
Yeast-Free White Rice Bread,
Egg Replacer, bulgur wheat,
Pure Soyquik, Nut Quik,
Pure Ricebran, Pure Rice Polish,
Corn Bran

Erewhon Products
U.S. Mills, Inc.
Omaha, NE 68111

nut butters, seed butters,
Barley Plus Oat Bran With
Toasted Wheat Germ,
Instant Oatmeal With Oat Bran

Fearn Natural Foods Division
of Modern Products, Inc.
P.O. Box 09398
Milwaukee, WI 53209

soya granules, soya powder,
baking mixes, pancake mixes,
corn germ, wheat germ

Food For Life Baking Co., Inc.
3580 Pasadena Avenue
Los Angeles, CA 90031

pasta,
muffins,
rice bread

G.M.B. Enterprises, Inc. Jersey City, NJ 07302	Goodman's Matzo meal
Garden of Eatin' Los Angeles, CA 90029	Blue Chips (blue corn chips)
Golden Temple P.O. Box 1802 Eugene, OR 97440-1802	whole grain cereals sweetened with fruit juice
Hain Pure Food Company, Inc. 13660 South Figueroa P.O. Box 5481 Terminal Annex Los Angeles, CA 90061	cold-pressed vegetable oils, rice cakes, large and mini home-style soups, home-style chili
Health Valley Foods 700 Union Street Montebello, CA 90640	natural cereals
Jackson-Mitchell, Inc. Turlock, CA 95381-0934	Meyenberg Powdered Goat Milk
Knudsen & Sons, Inc. Chico, CA 95926	natural fruit juices
Lakewood Products Miami, FL 33242	natural fruit juices, natural fruit drinks
Lifestream Natural Foods, Ltd. 12411 Vulcan Way Richmond, B.C. Canada V6V-1J7	Essene unleavened, sprouted grain breads
Lion Cross, Inc. North Bergen, NJ 07047	herb teas
Little Bear Organic Foods P.O. Box 682 Malibu, CA 90265	Bearitos Brand tortilla chips

Nature Food Centres
Wilmington, MA 01887

grains, herb teas,
chemical-free potato chips
and corn chips, pasta,
sea salt

Neshaminy Valley Natural
Foods
421 Pike Road
Huntingdon Valley, PA 19006

chickpea, millet, oat,
and quinoa flours,
soy and tofu powders,
rice cream, legumes, seeds,
grains, nuts, pasta

Niblack Foods, Inc.
Rochester, NY 14608

Bran-Gold Miller's Bran
and Wheat Germ

Ono Mills Co.
Mizusawa, Iwate Japan

white rice crackers

Pacific Rice Products, Inc.
Woodland, CA 95695

Apple Cinnamon Crispy
Cakes,
Brown Rice Hot Cereal

Parco Foods, Inc.
Blue Island, IL 60406

HOL*GRAIN Brown Rice Lite
Snack Thins

The Quaker Oats Company
P.O. Box 9003
Chicago, IL 60604-9003

rolled oats,
Mother's Oat Bran,
Mother's Quick Cooking Barley,
Mother's Rice Cakes,
Mother's Rolled Whole Wheat

Roman Meal Company
Consumer Services
P.O. Box 11126
Tacoma, WA 98411-0126

Wheat*Rye*Flax* 5-Minute
Cereal

Sandoz Nutrition
Minneapolis, MN 55416

Featherweight products:
sugar-free canned fruits,
low-sodium canned seafood,
salt-free juices,
cereal-free baking powder

Shaffer, Clarke & Co., Inc. Old Greenwich, CT 06870	WASA Lite Rye Crispbread, KA-ME Rice Crunch Crackers
Shiloh Farms, Inc. Box 97, Highway 59 Sulphur Springs, AR 72768	grains, organic flour, corn for popping, wheat flakes, rolled oats, legumes, meal, grits, wheat germ, bran, seeds, nuts, unsweetened, shredded coconut
Sovex Natural Foods, Inc. Collegedale, TN 37315	Good Shepherd Cereal sweetened with fruit juice, Oat Bran Hot Cereal
Spectrum Marketing, Inc. 133 Copeland Street Petaluma, CA 94952	cholesterol-free oils
Tom's of Maine, Inc. Kennebunkport, ME 04043	natural toothpaste, natural deodorant
Ventre Packing Co., Inc. Syracuse, NY 13204	Enrico's All Natural Spaghetti Sauce
Westbrae Natural Foods Emeryville, CA 94608	nut butters, tahini, unsweetened applesauce

CHAPTER SEVEN

The Breakfast Challenge

What grimmer prospect than lying in bed thinking about the day ahead without a clue in the world as to what to eat for breakfast. I've found myself in this hapless predicament on many a morning. Equally undesirable is finding oneself very hungry at mid-morning on a workday as a result of having eaten too little for breakfast. Knowing that lunch is another hour-and-a-half away can be disconcerting indeed. When this happens, I wish my body were a car so I could drive up to a pump, get fueled, and have the problem taken care of.

Breakfast requires a great deal of creativity on the Candida diet, and for this reason Candida patients ponder and discuss the subject frequently. Very often, when meeting another person on the diet, that person will ask, "What do you eat for breakfast? Please tell me!" Part of the problem is that we've been gastronomically programmed so that almost all the conventional choices for breakfast are very high in starch or contain yeast, sugar, chemicals, or a combination of these. A typical American breakfast consists of a glass of fruit juice, cereal with milk and sugar, eggs with toasted bread or bagels, or pancakes and bacon, or a danish pastry. All of these are usually accompanied by coffee or tea.

Another aspect of the breakfast dilemma is the fact that many people with Candida are plagued with numerous food allergies. And of course, among the most common allergens are the foods we eat regularly for breakfast: Coffee, tea, bread (which contains both wheat and baker's yeast), orange juice, eggs (yolk, white, or both), cow's milk, and sugar. As must be obvious by now, many of these foods are also generous providers of nourishment for the yeast-beast! What with eliminating both the allergenic no-nos and the yeast boosters from the breakfast menu, most Candida patients feel bereft of options. What to do?

Breakfast Suggestions

Being on the four-day rotation schedule in order to avoid developing more allergies has led some of the more clever Candida dieters to devise at least four breakfasts which are nutritious and allergen-free. This four-meal program can be repeated after the fourth day.

Those of you who tolerate eggs have a variety of options: On the day you choose to eat eggs, you could eat the usual egg dishes; or you could make an omelet, Chinese egg foo yong, eggs poached in stewed tomatoes, or corn custard. Other options might be a few small rice or barley pancakes, a half-waffle sweetened with orange or pineapple juice, whole wheat popovers, a slice of French toast made of homemade soy bread, or a homemade muffin, all of which contain eggs. A small portion of fried rice (either brown or white) made with beaten egg, in the oriental style, is another possibility. An allergy to egg yolk shouldn't stop you from making a "white omelet," using only egg whites and adding one or two of the usual fillings. On the other three days, you could choose to make egg-free pancakes, or muffins (buckwheat, for example), or a tofu shake sweetened with ripe banana, fresh peach, or mango. Still another idea is to have rice cakes or rye crackers, smeared with sunflower, almond, or sesame butter, or a small amount of plain butter. Well drained pork sausage (or sausage patties) with sautéed onions, shallots, or scallions is another possibility.

Cereals like oatmeal, cream of wheat, Wheatena, cream of rye, and cream of brown rice are all allowed on the diet, but do check the ingredients on all cereals, whether in a health food store (your best bet for cereals allowed on the diet) or a supermarket. One can also add a small amount of goat's milk, cow's milk (if you can tolerate it), or cream to sugar-free, malt-free cereals such as puffed rice, puffed millet, puffed corn, or puffed wheat. (El Molino and Health Valley make these.) Nature O's by Arrowhead Mills, a cereal that combines oat and white rice flours with defatted wheat germ is also recommended. Taking Amsnack Unsalted Brown Rice Chips, crumbling them, and adding milk is a novel idea; or take a rice cake (which can be easily found in supermarkets), crumble it, and add milk. A small amount of fresh fruit and/or a generous amount of nuts or seeds can also be added to any of these cereal dishes. If you must have a sweet taste and can tolerate the fruit sugar, put the milk (preferably goat's) in the blender with a fresh ripe peach, nectarine, mango, or banana before adding it to the cereal. Remember that you're better off using only half or one-third of a whole fruit so that fructose will be kept at a minimum. As another possible solution to the Candida breakfast dilemma, consider making yourself a regular meal, as the Japanese do. Imagine that it's lunchtime, and prepare a beef or veal patty accompanied by a vegetable like string beans, zucchini, or yellow summer squash. The nutrients in this type of breakfast will sustain you for several hours. Another suggestion is to heat up some soup made with a meat, chicken, or vegetable base which was prepared the day before or stored in the freezer. It's okay to add a small amount of lentils, kidney beans, or chick peas to these soups, as long as you're mindful of your daily carbohydrate intake.

The most foolproof way of avoiding unsatisfied early morning hunger is to *make sure you have the next day's breakfast food on hand when you go to bed at night.* These are some of the best words of advice I can give you. If you're coming home late at night and you know you need food for breakfast, stop at an all-night grocery store. Most towns around the country have at least one all-night store by now. Going to bed with no prospects on the breakfast horizon can only lead to going off the diet or going hungry.

Coffee is an important subject. Since the beans go through a drying process and often contain mold, coffee isn't recommended. Another consideration is that almost all coffees are gas-roasted, and many people with Candida react to the gas. Going without coffee, to which some people are addicted, is an adjustment to be made in your own way. But remember that dropping coffee (or tea) very suddenly can produce withdrawal symptoms, so it's advisable to wean yourself off them in this manner: Cut your intake to one half-cup each day for the first week, to one half-cup every other day for the second week, to one half-cup every third day for the next week, and, finally, to none at all.

As for tea, most of what's imported to the United States is black and fermented in order to produce a rich, flavorful brew. It, too, should be avoided, if you can wean yourself from it. As a substitute for morning tea or coffee, have one of the many wonderful decaffeinated herb teas, or Japanese green tea, which isn't fermented. Some people have tap water or spring water that's been boiled for ten minutes; others have boiled, diluted, fresh orange juice. Boiled water with fresh lemon juice is said to cleanse the body of toxins; this is also true of certain blood-purifying teas such as red clover blossom tea which can be bought in bulk at a health food store or an herb shop, such as the one in New York City called *Aphrodisia*. If you feel you absolutely can't go without coffee or tea in the morning, try continuing it at breakfast and see how it affects your progress on the diet.

Tofu is a great source of inspiration and creativity. For those of you who haven't been introduced, tofu is oriental soybean curd made by soaking soybeans, grinding them, and boiling the resulting purée. The soy milk that comes from straining the boiled purée is then curdled and put into boxes to form the finished product, a square, white cake. Tofu, which is used to nourish some of the world's underfed people today, has finally been recognized by the American public as an excellent source of protein which is not only high in calcium and phosphorus, but economical as well. It comes in both firm and soft textures and has a special talent for combining with herbs, spices, vegetables, meat, and seafood. It can be used with eggs, cheese and other milk products, and added to meat loaf.

How can tofu be used for breakfast? Try scrambling it with onions and eggs, or making tofu patties. Stir-fry tofu in slices with vegetables, or dip it in an egg batter, roll it in ground rolled oats (or pulverized rye crackers), and sauté it. If you can handle the fructose, make yourself a tofu "cocktail" (a tofu shake), by combining tofu with fresh fruit and fresh fruit juice in the blender. Some consider this a royal treat!

Those of you who eat breakfast in restaurants on a regular basis might wonder what to order. If you rotate your foods, you might order pork sausages on one day and eggs the next. You might have a few potatoes with one of those two dishes and, for the next day's choice, bring along some yeast-free brown rice or rye crackers, or one of your homemade muffins. Restaurant pancakes and waffles are ill-advised, even if eaten in small amounts, because they almost always contain sugar, and sometimes even yeast (in the enriched flour).

In a restaurant that serves meals all day, you could order, as the third day's breakfast choice, a burger without the bun, topped with sautéed onions and accompanied by a vegetable like string beans, carrots, zucchini, or whatever vegetables the menu offers. On the fourth day, you might have a half-grapefruit or a glass of fresh orange juice, followed by a bowl of cooked oatmeal. If you must have a dairy taste and can tolerate cow's milk, pour a little cream on the oatmeal. You might want to bring along some nuts to add variety and fiber to the oatmeal; you can also take them to work as a mid-morning snack. If you're not too vulnerable to fructose, one-half of a fruit like a pear or kiwi, or a slice of fresh pineapple, would also provide a mid-morning boost.

Making Breakfast a Treat

During the good weather season, Saturday is my favorite day to prepare breakfast. Even when I've gone to bed late on a Friday night, I rise early and eat a quick snack, knowing I will have breakfast later. Then I head up the sidewalk to the school playground on East 67th Street, the site of a large open-air farmers' market, called "Greenmarket," which is one of many such food fairs in New York City. The festive summer umbrellas shading the brightly-colored vegetables, bunches of marigolds and zinnias in orange and yellow, side-by-side with the pervasive, enticing aroma of fresh tarragon, thyme, and chives, all cast a spell on me. The abundant and fragrant perfumes of the shoppers can't hold a candle to the scent of fresh basil, which follows me through the market stalls. There's a hustle and bustle at the seafood stand and around the tables displaying vegetables, each shopper hoping to find the firmest yellow and brown peppers, the thinnest finger eggplants, and the perfect Kirby cucumbers. Inside the school building, not far away, there's the flea market, an array of picnic-style tables draped with shawls displaying all the charming handed- and re-handed-down flower vases, relish dishes, and egg cups one can take in. On the pavement, book vendors display their wares along stretches of fabric; on a lucky Saturday, I find at least one cookbook that inspires.

Arriving home from Greenmarket, I put my bounty in the fridge and begin to slice and sauté the delectable vegetables, freshly harvested from a New Jersey, Pennsylvania, or New York farm. This is in preparation for an omelet, a frittata (a round Italian-style omelet with no fold), or a side dish of vegetables to be served alongside a hunk of broiled sausage or a pair of home-made sausage patties.

I plan my rotated meals so that when Saturday comes, I can eat either eggs or sausage with vegetables from the farmers' market. One of my favorite combinations is fresh sausage with finely sliced yellow summer squash sautéed in vegetable oil with slivered carrots, shallots, and fresh tarragon. Sometimes I stir-fry a mélange of sliced okra rings, diced yellow wax beans, and slivered patty pan squash with scallions. For omelets and frittatas, I use a mixture of zucchini, onions, ripe tomatoes, and fresh dill; or I combine red peppers, shallots, thinly-sliced circles of finger eggplants, and fresh basil. When the rotating schedule tells me it's my day to eat rice, I'll add one of these vegetable combinations to cooked brown rice (leftover or newly prepared) and stir-fry the mixture with a beaten egg, substituting finely-chopped ginger root for the dill, tarragon, or basil.

Eight-Day Breakfast Plan for People on the Candida Diet

Here's a plan spanning eight days that can be followed or used for inspiration in designing your own breakfast plan. Rather than having to think about what to eat when you get up each morning, why not map out a plan for four days or more. It would certainly be helpful when shopping.

Day One
Zucchini and shallot omelet *or* two eggs any style. One half-cup mashed, boiled, or home fried potatoes *or* one homemade rice muffin.

Day Two
Fresh or frozen pork sausage (unsweetened and chemical-free) with string beans or yellow wax beans. Small bowl of cream of rye *or* two rye crackers *or* four or five Carr's Table Water Biscuits (made of wheat), spread with sunflower, sesame, or almond butter.

Day Three
One soy muffin (made with chopped apple or banana), eaten plain or with butter. One half-grapefruit, and nuts of your choice.

Day Four

Small bowl oatmeal *or* Nature O's cereal (with milk or cream) *or* an oat bran muffin. Broiled, well drained veal or beef patty with sautéed yellow summer squash or peppers or broiled tomato.

Day Five

Small portion of fried rice (preferably brown, for added nutrition) using oil of your choice with diced scallions, chives, or shallots, vegetables, shrimp (optional), and beaten egg using yolk, white, or whole egg (also optional).

Day Six

Small glass of fresh orange juice. Egg-free buckwheat pancakes with butter.

Day Seven

Tofu sautéed with onions and slivered carrots. Nuts of your choice.

Day Eight

Puffed wheat, puffed millet, or puffed corn with a small ripe peach, small nectarine, or one half-banana (with milk or cream). Ground lamb patty with fresh dill or rosemary and sautéed, slivered, fresh zucchini, string beans, or spinach.

Those of you on the Candida diet who have doctor's approval to eat fresh cheeses and yogurt may incorporate them into your breakfast menus. You can try mozzarella cheese (including the one made from buffalo milk), Canadian baby goat cheese, Swiss cheese (the one made in Switzerland), or processed American cheese melted on yeast-free crackers. Ricotta (made from cow's or goat's milk) can be tossed or blender mixed with a limited amount of fresh fruit such as peach, nectarine, pineapple, banana, apple, strawberries, or well washed, seedless white grapes (if tolerated). Or mix the same fruit with cottage or farmers cheese. Fresh goat cheese (*chevre frais* or Montrachet from France or Wisconsin) or regular cream cheese, blended or hand-mashed with the above-mentioned fruits, and topped with nuts and unsweetened, shredded coconut, makes another tasty treat. Yogurt made from cow's or goat's milk, or kefir, can be eaten plain or mixed with fresh fruit and topped with nuts and/or seeds.

Other Breakfast Suggestions for Candida Dieters

✓ Rice pudding (made with brown or white rice)

✓ Homemade jello (made of gelatin and fresh fruit juice)

✓ Stewed fresh fruit with cloves and cinnamon

✓ Whole wheat popovers with butter or cream cheese

✓ French toast (made with homemade rice bread or soy bread)

✓ Soybean milk shake (made in blender with fresh peach, nectarine, pear, mango, or banana)

✓ Tofu shake (made in blender with fresh fruit and fresh fruit juice)

✓ Lentil or vegetable soup (made with chicken, beef, or vegetable stock)

✓ Homemade hash

✓ Broiled pork chops (well drained of fat) with steamed vegetables

✓ Rice cakes or Soken's Vegetable Chips spread with sunflower, sesame, or almond butter

✓ Guacamole with yeast-free crackers

CHAPTER EIGHT

The Chinese Solution

One of the great pleasures in my daily life is lunching in Chinatown, which is a ten-minute walk from my office. New York's Chinatown is such a special world that going there for lunch is like going to another country. Walking up the incline of Mosco Street, I'm struck with the alluring, waffle-like aroma of Hong Kong egg cakes coming from an iron griddle in a tiny outdoor booth at the top of the hill. Sometimes there's a large group of people queued up, waiting for a cellophane bag of the plum-shaped cakes.

As I turn left or right at the top of the hill, I see the yellow and red façades of the shops with their vast array of dumplings, colored shrimp chips, pastries, and fire-engine-red bakery boxes. The china dishes, vases, and ornamental pieces from the Orient, masterworks of craftsmanship, force one to stop and look. Mott Street, as this charming and world-renowned street is called, is alive with Chinese residents, out-of-town tourists, and the multitudes of business people, jurors, judges, government workers, gourmets, and gourmands who come to Chinatown for a good lunch. Lining both sides of Mott are grocery stores, fish markets, bakeries, and produce stands displaying colorful mountains of fruit, eggplants, snow peas, water cress, broccoli, and all the exotic Chinese vegetables we Americans are finally discovering.

Chinese cuisine is one of the best choices you can make on the Candida diet, so try to find a good Chinese restaurant in your town or near your place of work. If you're familiar with Chinese cuisine, you know that many of the ingredients considered off limits for a Candida dieter and an allergenic are clearly absent from Chinese cooking. Chinese food is one of the most nutritious cuisines in that, for the most part, the ingredients are quickly stir-fried and retain most of their nutrients, juice, texture, and flavor. It also allows for maximum flexibility in making changes for Candida patients because almost all dishes are cooked to order. Except in the case of white rice (which one can elect to eat in small amounts), vitamins, minerals, and proteins are featured rather than carbohydrates. One would be hard pressed to find cheese, bread, or yeast in an authentic Chinese kitchen. The ginger, garlic, scallions, and onions commonly used as seasonings in Chinese dishes are fresh, and the oils polyunsaturated. Chinese chefs typically use a blend of vegetable oils or pure soybean oil.

Chinese Restaurant Dining

There's a tremendous variation in the quality of Chinese cooking, and for this reason I suggest you look for the restaurants offering simple, natural dishes that are free of fermentation, sugar, and complicated sauces. Equally important is finding a restaurant with a chef who's willing to be flexible in making a few adjustments. When I walk into some of my favorite haunts in Chinatown, the waiters go on automatic: As I'm sitting down at my table, they say, "Yes, I know: No soy sauce and no MSG." Depending on what I order, I sometimes add further instructions: "No black bean sauce" (Chinese-style black beans are fermented), or "No sugar and no cornstarch" (I'm allergic to corn). If I order squid with green and red peppers, for example, and don't specify otherwise, the dish will often arrive with black bean sauce and sometimes a touch of hot pepper spice or sugar or both. That's the way Chinatown restaurants in New York city normally prepare squid.

For those of you who have to avoid them, mushrooms are clearly the most difficult thing to get a Chinese chef to eliminate. Don't be surprised if a fungus such as a "tree ear" appears on your plate, even after you've requested that mushrooms be eliminated. The waiter will probably argue with you, saying "It's a fungus, not a mushroom!" If mushrooms are a no-no in your case, you might try saying that you're allergic to mushrooms and fungi and will get sick from eating them. These exchanges with waiters become easier if you keep going to the same restaurants; they'll eventually get to know your dietary needs and will explain them to the chef. One of the possible complications that may arise out of a request for "No soy sauce, no MSG, and no cornstarch" is that the waiter may bring out a dish that's steamed instead of stir-fried, often without salt as well. Therefore, it's wise to add at the end of your spiel, "But do sauté it with oil and add a little salt," (if you're allowed salt). I sometimes also add, "And it's okay to season it with garlic, ginger, scallions, or any combination of those." If the waiter speaks very little English or doesn't quite comprehend your request, find a diplomatic way of asking the manager to intervene.

As for Chinese tea, you'd better skip it because it's black tea and fermented, like most teas imported to the U.S. I usually accept the tea, pour a little into the cup, and let it sit there, because giving a waiter too many instructions can get complicated. Sometimes, at the outset, I take out my own herb tea bags and ask for a teapot filled with boiled water. Then there's the fortune cookie—it's a no-no because of the sugar, but Candida allows you to read the message, which, hopefully, will be an appropriate one like "Person who skips cookie will have big reward!"

MSG, or monosodium glutamate, is very commonly used in Chinese food. Many people complain of reactions after eating it, and get flushed or develop what some call a "Chinese headache." A Candida patient with food allergies should be aware that repeatedly eating foods with MSG could result in an MSG allergy. Another consideration is that MSG is commercially produced by the bacterial fermentation of sugar; in addition, it's high in sodium and, when used in combination with salt, can make a dish taste very salty.

The mustard and duck sauces that come in little dishes should be avoided because one has vinegar and the other sugar. You should also be aware that there's a difference between "roast pork" and "sliced pork" on Chinese menus. Opt for the sliced pork, because roast pork is usually coated with a barbecue sauce containing sugar.

Since this is a guide to diet rather than restaurants, I'm not going to recommend any particular Chinese restaurants, but I think I should give you some ideas of what to order when you're eating in one. Choosing a dish that contains a number of different vegetables like carrots, snow peas, peppers, tomatoes, baby corn, and onions all in the same dish isn't recommended if you're on the rotating diet, because you won't be able to have any of those things again for another four days. It's preferable to order like this: Shrimp with snow peas, broccoli, bean sprouts, or nuts (cashews or almonds); sliced fish with mixed Chinese vegetables (most of them you probably don't have at home or in non-Chinese restaurants, so it's okay to have a combination of them); or squid with mustard greens, peppers, or bean sprouts. Or you might have sliced pork with either string beans, Chinese broccoli (rapeseed), or snow peas; or beef with green pepper and onion; or beef with bean sprouts and scallion; or chicken combined with walnuts, cashews, or almonds, mixed Chinese vegetables, American broccoli, or snow peas.

When dining with several people, sautéed water cress, bean curd (tofu), snow peas, or stir-fried Chinese or American broccoli are all good vegetable dishes. Roast duck or crispy duck, without the sauce, and egg foo yong, with or without the mushrooms, are all good choices. Remember that the gravy that comes with egg foo yong doesn't usually have soy sauce in it. Hunan and Szechuan restaurants are more likely than Cantonese and Mandarin restaurants to feature soy sauce and sugar in their dishes. But since so many restaurants will deviate from their usual methods of cooking to accommodate you, why not try all the good restaurants, regardless of region.

One of the great advantages of Chinese restaurants in a big city like New York is that they're usually willing to take telephone orders and deliver food to your door. Those of you in smaller towns around the country can telephone your order and drive to the restaurant to pick up the hot food. You can transfer it to casserole dishes at home if you don't like paper containers. It's a quick, easy dinner for a family or a group of guests, Candida notwithstanding.

The Do-It-Yourself Alternative

If you live in a town where there are no Chinese restaurants, you can stir-fry your own Chinese dishes at home. Use a wok, an ordinary skillet, or a non-stick fry pan (providing you're not sensitive to the chemicals in non-stick pans) and choose an appropriate oil, such as soybean or walnut. By cooking in the Chinese style, you can also expand your vegetable horizons, which will give you more variety and serve you well if you're on the rotating diet. Chinese mustard greens, rapeseed broccoli, snow peas (fairly easy to find in supermarkets), kohlrabi, lotus root, Chinese cabbage, long purple eggplants, white eggplants, and fresh water chestnuts (you can peel them yourself) will all help to expand your repertoire for taste, nutrients, and choice. For a change of pace and added nutrition, make brown rice some of the time (for fried rice too); but remember to include the rice as part of your daily carbohydrate gram count. Chinese cooks usually use cornstarch when thickening sauces. If you have to avoid corn products because of sensitivities, use either arrowroot powder, rice flour, or potato starch as a thickener. Just remember that arrowroot loses its thickening powers when reheated. If you want to give dishes a more oriental flavor, add a little uncooked oriental sesame oil (available in Chinese supermarkets) just before serving.

Have you seen wonton and egg roll wrappers in the supermarket and wondered what to do with them? Most wontons and egg rolls served in Chinese restaurants have soy sauce in their fillings, but they needn't be off your list entirely, because if you're industrious or enjoy new cooking projects you can make wontons and egg rolls free of soy sauce at home. There are many inexpensive Chinese cookbooks in the stores, which describe how to make the fillings and explain the techniques of how to fold the dough. Freezing a batch of uncooked wontons and egg rolls to fry later should work out well. In the case of wontons, try simmering them in chicken or meat broth, either in their frozen or thawed states. Vegetables can be added to enhance the broth or they can be added to the soup simply to keep the wontons company. You and your family or friends can make an exhilarating group endeavor out of cooking Chinese food. Maybe you'll have some ideas of your own. There are endless possibilities.

Shopping for Chinese Products

If you aren't lucky enough to have a Chinese quarter like those in Boston, San Francisco, Los Angeles, New York, Washington, D.C., Chicago, Portland, Oregon, and Philadelphia (to name but a few), a large supermarket should have many of the ingredients used in oriental cooking. The local Chinatown markets usually have many fresh Chinese vegetables which are grown in the U.S. Chinese produce sold and consumed in New York City, for example, is grown on farms in nearby New Jersey in the summer, and in Florida all year round. In addition to shopping at the outdoor stands in Chinatown, you should go into the local Chinese supermarkets. Along with a marvelous array of vegetables, you'll find ginger root, bamboo shoots, fresh water chestnuts, and a large variety of unsalted, unprocessed nuts. Gravy thickeners like arrowroot and lotus root powders, rice vermicelli and soybean noodles (both great for people who can't tolerate wheat), egg noodles, oils, and a large selection of flours including white rice, sweet rice, sweet potato, soybean, and water chestnut all line the shelves.

Some oriental frozen foods, like ready-to-fry dumplings, are allowed on the diet, provided their contents don't include your allergens. Excellent fish markets are also to be found in the Chinese quarter, carrying items such as conch, smelts, and squid, which are less available elsewhere. Why not take home some of the less common types of seafood and expand your horizons there, too. Remember that seafood has iodine; iodine stimulates the thyroid, and the thyroid promotes mental alertness! You may also want to take home an uncooked duck. As you will see from the recipes, preparing it is much easier than you think and, in fact, will de-mystify duck roasting for you forever.

CHAPTER NINE

The Emergency Survival Kit

Recently, I took a weekend trip to a farm in Pennsylvania on the Amtrak train. On the way, I got hungry for a snack and went to the Café Car, only to find that there were only two things I could eat: Potato chips and soda water. I didn't want to eat potatoes, knowing I would probably be eating them over the weekend and that eating them now would interfere with the four-day rotating plan. I looked at the other Amtrak offerings: The nacho chips had cheese and preservatives; the cookies were filled with no-nos; the fruit juices were canned; the sandwiches had yeast; the donuts and the fruit sodas had sugar; coffee, tea, and wine were off limits; and hot dogs were out of the question! When I first began the Candida regime, this would have disheartened me, but, being a veteran, I opened my satchel and took out some toasted hazelnuts, a bag of unsweetened, shredded coconut, a washed pear, an herb tea bag, a small paring knife, and a paper plate. Using the airline-style table in front of me, I ate my snacks and drank the Café Car soda water with ice and a twist of lemon. Later on, I bought a cup of hot water and made herb tea. My companions, who were also on the Candida diet, had snacked on some homemade rice muffins and a container of fresh grapefruit juice, which they mixed with soda water from the Café Car.

When we arrived at our destination, a charming farmhouse where there were several other guests, snacks were served: Cheese, crackers, wine, and fresh apple cider. The cider was not apple juice; clearly, it was fermented. The crackers had yeast and sugar in them; and cheese and wine, need I say, were out of bounds. And so went the weekend: Vinegar in the salads, yeast in the bread, wine in the coq-au-vin, mold in the roquefort, fermented cheese in the quiche, and sugar in the fruit tart.

At first, thoughts of a two-day regimen of starvation ran through my mind and I began to get uneasy. Then I remembered my "Emergency Survival Kit," and went up to my room to find snack-packs containing yeast-free brown rice and rye crackers, Japanese potato snacks, toasted banana chips, pecans, and almonds. I'd also packed a lemon and a lime for salads, a small can of water-pack tuna, three different herb teas for three days, and a few fruits in case of dire famine. I'd been tipped off ahead of time that the farm was far from grocery outlets and the hostess wouldn't have time to take us shopping.

The three of us on the Candida diet were chided about our "odd" preoccupations about food several times during the weekend. We didn't bother to explain or justify them, because it wouldn't have helped. As the weekend went on, most of the guests got sick. A cold passed from person to person and, finally, to the hostess as well. Germs were abundant, probably because the guests, very young people, prepared food together, mostly without washing their hands. They sneezed everywhere, breathed on and touched each other. All the various ways colds are transmitted are still unclear, but they were certainly passed on that weekend—even though people slept dormitory style and didn't have sexual relations (to my knowledge).

The dénouement of this story is that all the guests left there with colds except for guess who? That's right, the three people with "odd eating habits." Our immune systems, after diet and treatment for Candida, were probably stronger than theirs. This was a great bonus.

Traveling long distance calls for advance planning, too. You can call the airlines ahead of time to order special food. Or you can opt to have a meal at home before leaving and bring snacks for the flight. Fresh fruit, potato chips, corn or brown rice chips, a few yeast-free crackers, and some nut butter or fresh cheese in a small plastic cup (with a spreader) are among the many possibilities.

Now that I've lost all reticence about bringing along my Candida diet goodies, I think nothing of taking out a box lunch on a trans-Atlantic flight. The last time I went to Paris, I brought much more than a box lunch with me. I used my carry-on case to pack all the vital emergency supplies, as well as a few small cans of unsmoked sardines and water-pack tuna with rip-off tops, a paring knife, and a vegetable peeler. The woman who cleaned my Paris hotel room probably thought I was a misplaced camper, but that's okay. I ate with the French in local restaurants at lunch and dinner, bringing along yeast-free crackers and my favorite herb teas (which I'd brought with me from the U.S. in case they weren't readily available in France). I'd ask for *"un pot d'eau chaude"* (a pot of hot water) and add my tea bag to it, as I did in all the local cafés. No French waiter or hotel room service thought a pot of hot water was a strange request.

I loved shopping for fruit, nuts, raw vegetables, goat cheese, and other snacks in the open air produce markets and local super-markets around the Rue de Seine (in St. Germain de Prés). Out-door markets abound in European cities and one can see the local townsfolk in one of their most colorful and natural habitats.

When shopping for food products in a foreign country, re-member to check labels for ingredients, as you would in your own country. It's also important to ask questions about how the food is prepared, when ordering in a foreign restaurant or café.

A list of key phrases in some of the more familiar foreign languages is included at the back of this book to aid you in asking for some of the essentials. This information can be supplemented with a small foreign-language booklet for travelers (Berlitz and others make them), which will help you get around with ease. Interaction with waiters and restaurant managers will probably make your trip more interesting and result in a few tales to take home.

With respect to diet food, traveling on an ocean liner or a cruise ship is usually an easier proposition because you're dealing with the same kitchen everyday. After a while they get used to making accommodations such as bringing lemon and oil for your salad and leaving the sweet sauce in the kitchen when you order roast duck. When packing for the ship, you'd do well to take the usual yeast-free crackers, snacks, herb tea bags, and other sup-plies, as you would when packing for a trip to Europe. Asking the waiter or cabin steward to store some fresh cheese (if allowed), a salad dressing you've brought with you, or medications that need refrigeration in the ship's galley or pantry, won't be seen as an outrageous request.

Those of you who travel within the United States for business purposes should be aware that some hotels offer rooms with kitch-enettes. In other circumstances, it's quite common to find a refrig-erator in the room or to have one brought in upon request, without charge or for a nominal fee. Inquire at the outset when reserving the room. With a fridge at your disposal, you can take along a homemade dressing for the salads which are usually available through room service, a few fresh cheeses (if allowed), and any other cold snacks you enjoy. If you don't have a fridge, you can still take your yeast-free crackers, nuts, nut butters, chips, sugar-free muffins, herb tea bags, medications, vitamins, and other supplies. Sometimes there's a grocery store nearby where you can pick up a few items. Most room service menus in American hotels offer tomato, orange, and grapefruit juices and sparkling water. Ice, which is usually on the house, is often dispensed by a nearby machine. I find that if I'm willing to make the effort to bring along the supplies that allow me to stay on the Candida diet, I can visit another city and be in top form the entire time I'm there.

I should add here that it's a good idea to have a small paring knife and a few paper napkins on you wherever you go, including in your own town, so you can pick up a piece of fruit, a carrot, an avocado, or something else if you feel overwhelmed by hunger. Carrying snack-packs (small plastic bags with nuts, seeds, chips, etc.) will help when hunger strikes. Business people who tote a briefcase can carry all sorts of things—wrapped, of course, so your kiwi fruit won't roll out during a Board of Directors' meeting.

This brings me to the workplace. Do you have a refrigerator at the office? If not, why don't you and a few co-workers pool your resources and buy one of the half-size units, which look like wood and blend in with the rest of the furniture. My office fridge is usually stocked with the following items: Bottles of sparkling water, a lemon, a lime, vegetable oil for lunches from the local salad bar, jars of nut butters, bags of nuts, crackers (which could become stale because they're free of preservatives), herb tea bags, medications that need to remain fresh, goat's milk, and goat cheese. Water-pack tuna, salmon, and sardines in tins, fresh fruit, hard-boiled eggs, and frozen homemade muffins (to be heated in the office microwave) are also in stock most of the time. My desk drawers store potato crackers, chips made from brown rice, seaweed, bananas, and carrots, and an abundant supply of vitamins.

Now to the hot pot. Since the office coffee machine is probably no longer of use to you, why not buy a hot pot for making herb tea with spring water (if the office supplies it) or plain tap water. You can also heat homemade soup in the hot pot, if you can't find a nearby restaurant that makes soup you can eat.

When there's an office party, you can bring some "legal" snacks for yourself and for the group, if you like, just in case the table is completely spread with no-nos. You might also bring along a bottle of one of your sugar-free, non-alcoholic drinks (see recipes), which other people may also want to sample, or pick up some seltzer or soda water if the party planner isn't willing. Shyness and reluctance about these matters can only stand in your way.

The Candida Patient's Everyday Survival Kit or S.O.S. Bag

Assembling a survival kit requires advance planning, creativity, and a sense of adventure. It's an area where your ingenuity and your own style come into play. On a day when you're bereft of ideas, consult the following list.

Food
✓ Raw vegetables: Celery, radishes, cucumbers, turnips, zucchini, cherry tomatoes, bell peppers, cauliflower, broccoli, carrots, and others of your choice;
✓ Hard-boiled egg;
✓ Crackers: Yeast-free rye, rice, or whole wheat matzo crackers, and rice cakes (large or mini-size) to accompany your lunches and restaurant meals (depending on how much starch you can tolerate);
✓ Nut and seed butters: Almond, sunflower, and sesame in small plastic container or glass jar;
✓ Nuts and seeds: Walnuts, pecans, hazelnuts, pine nuts, almonds, cashews (high in carbohydrates), sunflower seeds, and sesame seeds;
✓ Cheeses: Unfermented, only if allowed;
✓ Potato chips, chemical-free;
✓ Tortilla chips, chemical-free;
✓ Brown rice chips;
✓ Can of tuna, with rip-off top;
✓ Can of salmon;
✓ Can of sardines;
✓ Fruit (if allowed);
✓ One half-avocado.

Utensils
✓ Plastic knife, fork, and spoon;
✓ Small paring knife;
✓ Paper plate;
✓ Paper napkins;
✓ Small paper or plastic bag for refuse;
✓ Can opener, if needed.

Candida Food On-the-Go: Suggestions for Plane, Train, and Bus Trips

✓ Cold, broiled, or roasted chicken
✓ Sliced roast beef
✓ Sliced turkey, turkey loaf, or turkey meatballs
✓ Homemade meat loaf or meatballs (beef, veal, pork, or lamb)
✓ Cold sausage, chemical-free
✓ Cold shrimp with homemade lemon or lime mayonnaise
✓ Tuna salad with mayonnaise and yeast-free crackers
✓ Crab meat salad with mayonnaise and yeast-free crackers
✓ Chicken or turkey salad with mayonnaise and yeast-free crackers
✓ Container of Chinese restaurant food or homemade stir-fried dish
✓ Homemade soup or stew in a thermos
✓ Nuts and seeds
✓ Yeast-free rye or rice crackers, whole wheat matzo, or rice cakes with nut or seed butter
✓ Fresh cheeses (if allowed), with or without crackers. Use your creativity; some of them can be mixed with raw or cooked vegetables, chopped fresh herbs, fruit (if allowed), nuts, or fresh or canned seafood. Carry them in a plastic container, glass jar, or Chinese-style paper container.
✓ Fruit (if allowed)
✓ Any vegetable salad with allowed dressing
✓ Tossed salad from a salad bar with lemon and oil
✓ One half-avocado
✓ Celery stuffed with fresh cheese
✓ Black olives, American, not cured
✓ Guacamole with yeast-free crackers or tortilla, potato, or brown rice chips
✓ Yogurt dip (if allowed), with chips or crackers
✓ Cream cheese or fresh goat cheese dip (if allowed), with chips or crackers
✓ Tofu-avocado dip, with chips or crackers

✓ Tofu "cocktail" (see recipes) in a thermos
✓ Fresh orange or grapefruit juice, diluted
✓ Fresh fruit juice to add to sparkling water (for planes and trains)
✓ Herb tea bags (for planes and trains)
✓ Iced herb tea in a thermos.

CHAPTER TEN

Socializing on the Candida Diet

Eating out, visiting friends, and entertaining at home are all important for people in treatment for Candida. While it's true that you're more limited than before, accepting the diet as an alteration of your *gastronomic* lifestyle, and not as an alteration of your *total* lifestyle, will probably bear fruits for you. Those of you who are gourmets and gourmet cooks can continue to enjoy food. You can do plenty of cooking and eating, providing you choose the right ingredients and prepare them according to the guidelines of the Candida diet. There's no reason to stay away from your local cafés and restaurants—what changes is what you order and, in some cases, how it's prepared. It's also important to consider that not all your social activities have to be centered around food and drink. With the same people you might ordinarily meet for a meal, you can take a walk in the park, go to the health club, take a drive in the country, or plan some other entertainment. Movies, for example, have no yeast.

Going out to Dinner

Eating in a restaurant is easier than you might imagine. After a while, you'll know which restaurants have waiters, chefs, and managers who are willing to make a few accommodations. Familiarizing yourself with menus will let you know where you can find good food that's free of vinegar, sugar, wine sauces, and other no-nos.

Remember, you can have broiled, roasted, baked, or sautéed food that's prepared with oil or butter. When ordering fish, ask to be spared the paprika sprinkled on top because it's a dried spice and may not be cooked enough to kill any mold. Oil and lemon on the side are recommended with salad, or you may want to bring your own salad dressing or homemade mayonnaise.

There are a couple of questions I try to remember to ask waiters in restaurants. One is: "Do the carrots have sugar added to them?" Another is: "Is the dish served with a sauce on it?" If so, I ask the waiter to eliminate the sauce or serve it on the side, depending on what's in it. This is especially necessary with roast duckling, since most sauces that accompany duck contain sugar and, in many cases, alcohol. With an omelet, you can ask them to leave out the cheese (unless it's allowed) and, in the case of scrambled eggs, to leave out the milk, if they happen to use it (and if you're allergic to it). If you react to wheat, flour-thickened gravies are hazardous and it's wise to prevail upon the waiter to find out what was used as a thickener. Sometimes, as is probable with roast beef, there's no flour added and the meat arrives resting on a sea of natural juice. Ask questions!

You can order soda water or some other sparkling water with lemon or lime for a beverage, both before and after your meal. Fresh strawberries or a half-grapefruit can serve as dessert; or you can hold off for a homemade dessert later. If it's a very "relaxed" restaurant, you can bring along a couple of homemade, sugar-free cookies. When leaving the restaurant, it's a good idea to thank the waiter or waitress for accommodating you and, if you can, leave a little extra tip. Explaining to the manager that you like his place because it's more flexible than other restaurants will probably work wonders the next time you come in. In the case of a restaurant near work that you visit frequently, getting to know the manager is recommended. The sooner they learn your dietary requirements, the better for you.

Some restaurant cuisines serve your needs better than others. Generally speaking, the more simple the cooking, the better. French food in the classic tradition is bound to be prepared with ingredients that don't serve your purposes. The traditional method of French cooking with heavy sauces evolved because at one time in French history, food traveled long distances and was not very fresh on arrival. French cooks employed heavy-handed seasonings and sauces as a way of disguising the lack of freshness. The French nouvelle cuisine of today is much more health conscious and suitable to our modern lifestyle.

Chinese cooking lends itself to the Candida diet better than any other ethnic cuisine, as mentioned earlier. Fortunately, Greek and Italian cuisines also lend themselves to the Candida diet. In the case of Italian cuisine, the meat, fowl, fish, and vegetable dishes are very suitable. Although most pasta has no yeast, it's high in simple carbohydrates and your intake should be governed by how much starch you can handle. As mentioned previously, whole wheat pasta is recommended over white flour pasta. On the other hand, veal piccata, chicken with rosemary, fish or scampi with lemon butter, homemade soups (if they don't contain your allergens), sautéed vegetables, and salads with lemon and oil are all good choices. In the case of a dish like veal piccata, which is usually made with wheat flour, you can ask to have the flour eliminated if you react to wheat. A side order of rice can accompany the dish as one of the vegetables if you can't get two low carbohydrate vegetables. This choice, too, should depend on your capacity to handle carbohydrates. Sometimes a double order of an unstarchy vegetable like spinach, escarole, zucchini, string beans, or broccoli is the best choice.

In a Greek restaurant, egg-lemon soup, hummos (a mashed chickpea spread), or stuffed grape leaves (containing white rice and seasonings) can be ordered as appetizers. If you have to avoid canned goods at all costs, stay away from stuffed grape leaves, because the grape leaves served in restaurants and salad bars are usually canned. As a main course, you can opt for lamb shish kebab skewered with vegetables, served with a small portion of rice or a large portion of vegetables. Or you might choose one of the shrimp entrées. These dishes will probably be accompanied by a Greek salad, which you should have without the feta cheese or cured black olives because they're fermented. The Greeks often use lemon juice instead of vinegar in their cooking, but do ask what's in the shish kebab marinade and make sure that no vinegar is used in the salad. Greek menus frequently include roast leg of lamb, broiled chicken, grilled pork chops, and gyros, a seasoned meat loaf cooked on a vertical rotisserie. These are all good choices. If you react to tomatoes, be sure to ask the waiter, at the outset, to refrain from topping your dish with tomato sauce, a common practice in Greek restaurants.

You'll fare quite well in a Mexican restaurant if you can eat corn, because taco shells and tortilla chips are made of stone-ground corn. You can have guacamole, tacos, and tostadas without the cheese and sour cream. If you can handle the carbohydrates, you can have a very small portion of rice and refried beans along with a salad dressed with lemon and oil. There may also be chicken and shrimp entrées on the menu, accompanied by rice. When asking that certain ingredients (like cheese and sour cream) be omitted from the dishes of your choice, bear in mind that waiters and chefs don't always follow instructions. One way to guarantee success is to say that these additions will make you sick.

Many people find themselves in fast food establishments on a no-cooking night. There are certain choices there too. In a place serving fried chicken made with a batter of bread crumbs rather than flour, it's advisable to peel off the crumbs. Be aware that almost all the flour used in flour batter is made from wheat, and some of it is fortified with yeast. There are french fries in such restaurants, but you must eat them in limited numbers because of the carbohydrates and for other health reasons. Restaurant-made cole slaw usually contains vinegar and sugar, so it's on the no-no list. In a hamburger restaurant, you might order a hamburger without the bun, a handful of fries, and if available, lettuce and tomatoes with raw onions. Skip the ketchup, which has sugar and vinegar in it, and if you need a topping, bring your own home-made mayonnaise.

Visiting Friends

Eating at someone else's house isn't as easy as going to a restaurant, because you usually don't have a choice of food. It's best to call the host(ess) ahead and give a short explanation of your dietary needs. Outlining in detail what you *cannot* eat will only leave the person at the other end bewildered as to what to cook. A concise, reasonable explanation of what you *can* have might go something like this:

> I eat broiled, boiled, or roasted meat, chicken, and seafood except for (cite allergens) as long as there are no bread crumbs used. Then all vegetables except for (cite vegetable allergens). I have lemon or lime and oil on my salad rather than vinegar. Instead of bread, I eat potatoes or rice (if, in fact, you do). For dessert, I usually have a piece of fruit (if you're allowed fruit), such as (cite a few examples). To drink, the best things would be sparkling water and herb tea. And could I ask you to spare the (specify any other allergens here, like wheat, corn, tomatoes, milk, cinnamon, and so forth)?

You might want to offer to bring something for the meal, like a salad dressing for the group or for yourself and/or something for dessert like cut-up fresh fruit or a sugarless quickbread along with your herb tea bags. If household animals give you an allergic reaction, you'd better mention that too.

In the case of an invitation that won't allow for special requests, like an invitation to a sit-down dinner or buffet for a large group, you could elect to eat before you go, and nibble during the meal. I know someone who, when unable to find anything to eat at a dinner, says she's having medical tests the next day and must fast for the next twelve hours. To find nothing at all to eat at a gathering is rare on the Candida diet.

On those occasions when I'm out socially and asked why I'm not eating everything, I sometimes say: "I'm having a problem with yeast and have to avoid certain foods for a while." Very few people pursue this explanation since it isn't very intriguing. The explanation that "I have a condition called chronic candidiasis and have to stay on a diet" provokes too much curiosity. Another way I get off the hook is to tell people I've developed some allergies and have to avoid certain foods. I never say anything that's not true!

If the invitation is to a very small gathering and you know the cook in question will prepare fancy, highly-sauced food no matter what, you can go and hope for the best, or you can find some foolproof way of turning down the invitation. Declining is highly recommended in the case of an invitation to spend several days at the home of someone you know wouldn't adjust the menu if the Queen of England were coming. There are many folks who think that allergies are "all in the head." Beware of such people, if you have allergies, because, thinking it's all nonsense, they might add your allergens to the pot anyway. My way of reprogramming people who think that way is to let them know that it's possible to die from an allergic reaction!

When planning a visit to someone's house in the country for the weekend, it's best to explain, when first invited, that you're on a yeast-free, sugar-free diet and there are many foods you can't eat. The host(ess) will probably ask what that means and you can go into the explanation of what you *can* eat, as described earlier. I usually ask if he or she would be offended if I brought along a few of my diet supplies. If you recall the tale of my weekend in the Pennsylvania farmhouse, I travel fairly well supplied if I expect that there won't be too much Candida diet food in the offing.

Having a car for the weekend facilitates skipping off to the nearest market or restaurant when you're hungry. The Pennsylvania weekend was a good exercise in how to handle a situation in which the kitchen can't be very flexible because of the number of guests, and going to a supermarket is not an option.

Almost every kitchen anticipating guests has eggs, onions, potatoes, and salad vegetables. It's wise, then, to bring along some of the special items you might need, like yeast-free crackers, malt-free cereal, goat's milk (if necessary), and a few bags of the particular herb teas you drink. You should also pack the usual snacks and a homemade salad dressing or a lemon or lime for your salads.

Entertaining at Home

Entertaining at home is the easiest way to socialize on the Candida diet; you simply make the dishes *you* can eat for your guests. You can say it's food related to your diet or you can choose to say nothing, because there's no way of telling the difference between "Candida food" and regular food. Except for the absence of bread and the offering of sugarless pastry, there are no clues. When I serve some of the sugarless quickbreads I make (banana, pumpkin, cranberry, prune, or apple), people usually say they like them or they don't comment. Some of them may think it's a low-calorie concept. I have no qualms about telling guests they're going to eat food from a diet they've never been on, and, as a result, go home feeling better than when they came. Offering them wine, brandy, coffee, and whatever else they want to drink while I have Candida drinks and herb tea, works out very well.

Throwing a cocktail party is one of the simpler ways of socializing at home. You can give guests whatever they like to drink while you have seltzer or fresh juice with seltzer and a slice of lemon or lime. Consult the recipes for tofu "cocktails" and other delicious drinks.

There are endless possibilities for snacks and finger food. Aside from nuts, you can serve guacamole, paté, tuna-mayo spread, or some creative tofu mixture on toasted sourdough rye bread triangles or yeast-free crackers. Other choices might be lamb, veal, or turkey meatballs, and cold hunks of sausage on toothpicks. Deviled eggs made of lemon or lime mayonnaise mixed with crab meat and fresh herbs (like basil or dill) is another possibility. Cruditées (assorted cut-up raw vegetables) or chips made from brown rice, carrot, potato, sea vegetables, or corn (all found at the health food store) can be accompanied by avocado, mashed bean, anchovy, caviar, salmon, crab meat, or clam dip made with homemade mayonnaise. Or substitute cream cheese, fresh goat cheese, or yogurt for the mayonnaise in these dips. Fruits (like pineapple, peaches, or tart apples), cut in chunks and speared with toothpicks, are good by themselves or served around a dipping bowl of homemade mayonnaise blended with straw-berries, banana, or avocado (with tofu added, if you like). Chopped almonds, pecans, or walnuts can also be added to the mayonnaise-and-fruit mixture. People who can eat fresh cheeses can blend strawberries, pineapple, banana, avocado, or mango with cottage cheese, cream cheese, or fresh goat cheese to use as a spread with crackers. The cocktail party is highly recommended when entertaining because you can minimize the labor, do a great deal of the preparation in advance, and skip the work in-volved with dessert and coffee.

When having guests for dinner, you can serve any of the cock-tail snacks above with drinks. Consider some of the following suggestions for meals. Serve shrimp broiled with oil or butter, parsley, fresh garlic, and shallots with a green vegetable and a starch, like brown rice, barley, potatoes, or butternut squash. Or consider as a main course roast pork with onions and carrots cooked alongside. This could be accompanied by a sugarless ap-plesauce (Mott's and other companies make it, or you can make your own) or a slice of broiled pineapple. Roast duck with pineap-ple sauce is enticing. Parsnips or brown, wild, or wehani rice (a dark brown California rice found in health food stores) and string beans could accompany the duck. Peas and yellow summer squash with no rice might be another option, or you might serve a small portion of one of the orange winter squashes with broc-coli or zucchini. A baked fish from fresh or salt water, stuffed with a crumbled yeast-free cracker dressing, or broiled scallops (fresh or frozen) served with two low-carbohydrate vegetables would also make a nice main course.

Poultry has endless possibilities. Chicken can be prepared with a fresh lemon, lime, or orange sauce, or with fresh or dried spices tucked under its skin before broiling. There's also chicken cacciatore, using rosemary, lemon juice (instead of wine), onions, and small pieces of carrots instead of tomatoes (if you or your guests react to tomatoes). You can also stir-fry sliced, boneless chicken with vegetables and serve them with or without rice. Adding a few drops of uncooked sesame oil (the type found in oriental markets) can give this dish a more exotic flavor.

A dinner of roast turkey stuffed with a dressing made of broken-up Wasa Lite rye crackers, or with cooked rice or barley, or a stuffing made of rolled oats, onions, pine nuts, fresh red pepper, sage, and other seasonings (as outlined in the recipes) almost guarantees an enthusiastic response. I recently served roast chicken made with a rolled oats stuffing to someone who thought it was delicious and didn't even notice the absence of bread. The same stuffing could be made with barley flakes (from the health food store), which are the barley counterpart to rolled oats. If the guests must have something sweet, as a substitute for cranberry sauce you can serve pears baked with nutmeg or fresh pineapple broiled with cinnamon and a little butter or oil.

Baby cornish hens stuffed with a mixture of wild rice, shallots, nuts served with gravy laced with fresh orange juice and dill and thickened with barley, rice, or whole wheat flour is an enticing idea. You might want to try stuffing the hens with brown or white rice mixed with sautéed leeks, diced fresh pineapple, and toasted pecans.

You'll probably love using the whole range of today's vegetables found in supermarkets, produce, and farmers markets. Why not plunge in and try them all, since diversity is in order on the Candida diet? Kohlrabi, white eggplant (remove the tough skin), peppers of all colors, escarole, kale, okra, beets, artichokes, snow peas, water chestnuts, lima beans, leeks,and wax beans (butter beans) are all interesting. Then there's Chinese rapeseed, broccoli, lotus root, bean sprouts, red cabbage, Brussels sprouts, endive, fennel, Swiss chard, yellow turnips (rutabagas), vidalia onions, red onions, shallots, and yellow tomatoes. All of these plus the full range of squashes (including patty pan, acorn, buttercup, spaghetti, Hubbard, dumpling, and pumpkin) should make for a delightful and healthy eating adventure.

A suitable salad might be water cress with sliced, peeled oranges and lemon mayonnaise (or just plain extra virgin olive oil), topped with slivered nuts. Or serve a plain green salad with lime juice, oil, and fresh basil (or dill), or a tahini dressing (see recipes). Other possibilities for salad might be arugula, water cress, radicchio (a red Italian lettuce), or a combination of these tossed with Chinese sesame oil or plain hazelnut oil (found in gourmet and specialty shops) and topped with pine nuts.

Serving your guests certain foods such as garlic bread and fermented cheeses with the meal will probably please them. But if you know you don't have the will power to pass on these, you'd best not serve them.

For dessert, you can always serve a colorful platter of sliced, fresh fruit, plain or with Banana Whipped Cream (or ricotta cheese, if allowed), and chopped nuts on the side. Dessert should not present a problem because the recipes in this book contain a number of ideas for quickbreads, cakes, pies, and other desserts sure to please even the non-Candida palate.

The Decorative Touches

The decoration of both house and table can enhance a meal tremendously. You can serve the most modest spread, garnished inexpensively but creatively, and people will think it's wonderful. I've seen the most costly, labor-intensive food served in a dull fashion and the response has been just as dull.

If you or the guests are sensitive to fumes from candles, eliminate them and feature flowers, fruit, or a combination of both. Decorating the table colorfully with flowers or fruit influences the mood of the guests. There is no end to how elaborate you can be with fresh flowers, but if economy is a high priority, you can use something you can eat later, like three oranges or eight or nine plums arranged on a bed of leaves you've picked yourself. Balloons in clusters around the room are super economical and very festive. Some party shops, and many florists, sell individual helium balloons that will keep their buoyancy for hours. Paper flowers can be used over and over, but keep them free of dust.

Fresh flowers are possible, even on a low budget. Using a pot full of leaves from the garden or the flower shop, you can add just three or four flowers for a table centerpiece. In the summer, outside the cities, you can use tree, shrub, and ground cover greens from the garden and Queen Anne's lace and wild daisies which grow abundantly along the highways. In places like Massachusetts and Connecticut, it's possible to find wild roses and orange day lilies (the blooms last one day) growing along country roads. Just remember to make the floral centerpieces low enough in height so that guests can see each other. If you're at all artistically inclined, decorating food platters with radish flowers, carrot swirls, scallion brushes, baby tomatoes, black olives, lemon, lime, or orange slices, parsley, or water cress adds aesthetic appeal. There are lots of books and tools available for decorating food. This art form, by the way, is known as *"garde-manger,"* a term borrowed from the French. If you're willing to unleash your creativity, you can have boundless fun developing your skills at this.

Picnics and Boat Rides

Going on a picnic or a boat ride for which you're in charge of either organizing or preparing the spread can be another safe way of socializing and staying on the Candida diet. Once again, there's no reason for the others to know it's a diet menu.

Among the many interesting choices for a picnic spread or for the ship's deck are raw vegetables with a guacamole, mayonnaise, tofu, or yogurt dip, seafood salads with homemade mayonnaise, Candida-style southern fried chicken (see recipes), cold tarragon chicken, meatballs, meat loaf, cold sausage, and French-style patés. Good choices for dessert are fresh fruit, or something baked, like apricot-oat squares, banana spice cake, banana ball cookies, or oatmeal cookies, for all of which there are recipes in this book. Adding cheese, wine, beer, and regular pastry for people who can have them is a fine idea (providing *you* can resist). When I go on a picnic with people who don't have Candida, they often ask for suggestions for treats on the diet that they can bring. Some people are extremely sympathetic and considerate of your situation, while others can be quite the opposite. You'll learn a great deal about your friends, relatives, and spouse while on this diet.

The Candida Gourmet Society

Now let's talk about organizing a new group. Have you ever heard of the *Candida Gourmet Society?* I have, because I created it. It's a group of people who get together to socialize, dine, lunch, or brunch together, in the Candida style. Finding members is usually accomplished by putting a notice in the classified ads of the local newspapers or asking doctors to recommend possible candidates. Some groups post notices on community bulletin boards or in health clubs, or they simply ask around. Often, people who work in health food stores know customers who have Candida.

When organizing a gourmet society, you may want to indicate

in your notices that while it isn't necessary to be a gourmet to attend a meeting of the Candida Gourmet Society, it *is* necessary to be on the Candida diet. Get-togethers of the gourmet group not only provide emotional support, they usually include talk of new culinary creations by members and new recipes from books and magazines which can be used intact or can be adapted to the Candida style of cooking. Sometimes people bring samples for the rest of the group—a new muffin, cookie, or quickbread they've made, or a Candida kosher snack they've found in the shops.

Conversation can center around any number of topics and can be dictated by the particular personalities in the group. For instance, if you had Arthur Miller, Henry Kissinger, and Billie Jean King in your group (I have no actual knowledge of their health), I don't think you'd want to spend the whole evening discussing the fungicidal capacity of Amphotericin-B or the pros and cons of eating calf's liver. Why not capitalize on what the members have to offer?

Your group may want to celebrate holidays like Christmas and Thanksgiving, and organize picnics, fishing trips, tailgate parties, boat rides, and ski trips (for the almost well). If you decide to convene on each other's birthdays, there's an orange-pecan birthday cake in the recipe section which can be served with "legal" drinks or herb tea.

The group can elect to meet in a restaurant where the food is certain to be properly prepared, and perhaps even ordered ahead. Or the regular get-togethers can be done on an alternating basis, that is, at a different house each time. If you meet at someone's home, the entire dinner can be prepared by the host(ess), or it can be a group endeavor where each person is responsible for a particular dish. An alternative would be to serve a buffet with a variety of dishes. Consulting with each other ahead of time about the menu is advisable so that people on the four-day rotating diet can refrain from eating the foods to be served during the three-day-period before you meet. Allergies that may be pervasive in the group, such as cow's milk, wheat, and corn, should be taken into account.

Planning a buffet incorporating the idea of rotating foods on an every-fourth-day basis merits consideration. You could take two main courses, like chicken and pork, or shrimp and beef, and encourage members to create something using those two foods as featured ingredients so they won't use up all their food options in one meal. If some members are not culinarily inclined, give them a recipe and offer help over the phone.

If shrimp and beef, for example, are to be the primary ingredients for a meal (assuming no members are allergic to both), you could create a menu consisting of shrimp salad, batter-fried shrimp, shrimp and stir-fried vegetables (served hot or cold), shrimp curry, a shrimp and rice casserole (like Chinese fried rice and shrimp without the soy sauce), or a shrimp frittata in the case of brunch.

Using beef as the other featured food, you could have beef stew and a bowl of sliced, cold roast beef with fresh dill (or tarragon) mayonnaise tossed with a salad of Boston lettuce, scallions, cucumbers, dill, and parsley. Meat loaf minus egg and wheat flour (if people are allergic to these), meatballs, and curried ground beef with peas and onions would all work well. To accompany the beef and shrimp dishes, you could select from a variety of vegetable salads using non-vinegar dressings. Centering a meal around pork and crab meat, or around a combination of lamb and turkey on another occasion, would almost certainly spark people's creativity.

The idea of forming a Candida Gourmet Society not only makes life more pleasant when you're dealing with a diet and a health problem, it brings new opportunities for expanding your social and intellectual horizons. You know at the outset that you'll have at least three meeting grounds with the new people: You're all members of the human race, you're all in treatment for the same illness, and you're all on a similar diet. It's a concept worthy of exploration; at worst, it will be an interesting experiment and, at best, a great deal of fun.

The Family Situation

In a family situation, one or more than one person may have Candida. The person cooking can choose to prepare a special meal for the people affected, or to prepare a Candida meal for the entire family, since the diet is so varied and healthy. Preparing a Candida meal and adding a few bread rolls (with yeast) and perhaps a more conventional dessert for the family members who aren't affected is okay. However, teaching your family to give up desserts containing sugar altogether is something to consider. If the family member who cooks doesn't have Candida, then he or she should study the diet carefully or actually go on it for a while in order to fully understand it. That person will have nothing to lose but poor eating habits and pounds!

It would be preferable that the person most familiar with the diet, and most meticulous about reading labels and looking for fresh produce, do the shopping. This should not be someone short on time and patience, since shopping requires traveling to more than one location. Some supermarkets, like the Heartland Food Warehouse in New England, have almost everything under one roof, including a substantial amount of health food; but going to a health food store for some of the Candida kosher crackers, flours, and oils will probably still be necessary.

How members of your family deal with your situation is important. Hopefully, they'll have some compassion and won't ridicule or complain about your situation. Friends and relatives can create problems, since many of them may not be sufficiently familiar with Candida and may be quick to label it a "fictitious illness" or another contemporary fad. Would that Candida would go out of style!

One way you might cope with those close to you, if they're making life difficult, is to tell them that the diet is something you *have to do* so you can live your life and function normally again. You might suggest that if they're going to give you a hard time while you're on the diet, perhaps it's best that you see them again after the problem is conquered, which could be a way down the road. This approach won't work with people who live in the same household with you, but it might work well with friends and relatives, regardless of how they may feel about the legitimacy of Candida. As for people sharing the same living space, it's probably necessary to sit down and have a serious talk with anyone who's creating a problem. Perhaps that person can read some of the key chapters in this book.

Those of you who have a sexual partner should be aware that Candida can be sexually transmittable. The more genetically predisposed and the more immune-compromised the unaffected partner, the greater the possibility that Candida may be transmitted. A woman giving Candida to a man is the more likely scenario. Women are more likely to have Candida because of the difference in their hormonal makeup and because the vagina provides a warm, moist setting for yeast organisms to proliferate. In addition, women are more attentive to their health problems than men are, and more likely therefore to have had a few too many rounds of antibiotics. Another of life's ironies!

You'll have to deal with the possibility of transmitting this illness to another person and resolve it with your partner in your own way. Bear in mind that a person who develops Candida can have an immune system weak enough to make cancer, arthritis, AIDS, and a host of other diseases more threatening. While this is more of a possibility in cases of *untreated* individuals, I feel I should make you aware of all the implications of having Candida.

Smoking

Another domestic matter to be considered is the problem of smoking. Not only do most people who have Candida react unfavorably to smoke, it facilitates the growth of yeast. People who have Candida and continue to smoke are aggravating the situation. As you know, getting someone to give up smoking is similar to dealing with an alcoholic—*they* will decide when to stop. You may want to make a rule in your home that all smoking take place in the basement, the garage, or outdoors. I don't allow people to smoke in my apartment anymore, and while some of them don't like it, they do go along with smoking in the area of the stairwell down the hall.

Support Groups

In many cities, like New York, there are Candida support groups which are either chapters of an organization called the Human Ecology Action League (H.E.A.L.) or independent support groups which have evolved on their own. I used to go to a group in which people talked about their Candida-related problems, reported on their progress, discussed any new information they had uncovered, gave accounts of what they'd been eating, and generally provided emotional support. Sometimes members would say they'd had a stint off the diet and would describe reactions. At other times, they might compare notes on the various aspects of their doctors' treatment. Comparing notes on doctors can be extremely helpful, because each doctor's way of dealing with Candida can be quite different. Someone else's doctor may practice a form of treatment you can suggest to your own doctor. It's also possible to get from the group the supportive relationship you may not be getting elsewhere. If a support group doesn't exist in your town, you could go about recruiting members and organizing one in much the same way you would organize a Candida Gourmet Society.

Wishing You Well

Now that I've indoctrinated you into all the aspects of the Candida diet lifestyle, and shared everything but my long toiled-over recipes (which are coming up next), I think it's time to say "Good luck" and to tell you, just in case you don't know, that I'm rooting for you all the way!

CHAPTER ELEVEN

The Recipes

As you'll see, I've developed an abundance of high fructose beverages and high carbohydrate breads, muffins, waffles, and desserts. This is not because I want to nourish your Candida; it's because a person on a diet which excludes yeast, sugar, honey and, in many cases, cow's milk, wheat, and gluten, will have to go without commercially-made beverages, breads, muffins, waffles, and desserts almost all the time. The best approach for a person on the Candida diet is to include the high carbohydrate, high fructose recipes in your regimen, *in small portions* at first, to see how you fare. If you feel much better without them, perhaps they should be reserved for special occasions and for holiday meals, or avoided altogether.

Most of the recipes for main courses and salads in this section are intended to be used as everyday fare, not only for you, but for family and guests. I haven't included too many vegetable recipes, although they're a very important component of the Candida diet, because they're easy to do.

The book provides an ample supply of recipes as a way of showing you how to prepare Candida food that's interesting, flavorful, and nutritious. I also want to inspire you to come up with your own ideas. Many of the dishes referred to in the text of the book can be found in this section. The flour substitution chart and the corn-free baking powder recipe are included for those who have problems with gluten and/or with grains such as wheat and corn. As you'll see, there's no reason for a Candida or an allergy patient to be deprived of the great pleasure of dining well.

APPETIZERS

Avocado-Crab Appetizer

Ingredients
1 standard-size ripe avocado, peeled
Homemade mayonnaise or blender mayonnaise to taste
1 6-oz. can white crab meat, well drained
Fresh parsley
Fresh basil or dill (optional)
Salt (optional)
Boston (butter) lettuce and vegetables of your choice for garnish
Chemical-free potato chips for dipping (optional)

Method
1. In soup plate, mash avocado with mayonnaise, using fork.
2. Add crab meat and blend well into mixture.
3. Wash, dry, and chop fresh parsley and fresh basil or dill, adding as much as suits your taste. Add salt, if allowed, and blend thoroughly. Cover with plastic wrap and chill.
4. Arrange mixture on washed and drained Boston (butter) lettuce leaves with vegetable garnishes, such as carrot circles, red pepper rings, and black olives or garnishes of your choice. Serve potato chips alongside.
   Yield: 2 ample servings.
   Note: Serve as appetizer before meal or on toasted rice cake as snack any time of day. Also good on crackers with "cocktails" before dinner. Add finely-chopped celery, if desired. Buy a second avocado for this recipe, in case the first is flavorless.

Guacamole

Ingredients
½ teaspoon minced fresh garlic
1 tablespoon freshly squeezed lemon or lime juice
¼ teaspoon salt, if allowed
1 standard-size avocado, peeled and cut
Tortilla chips, chemical-free potato chips or raw vegetables for dipping

Method

1. Put garlic, juice, and salt in blender jar; chop, blend, and purée.
2. Add avocado and chop, blend, and purée until completely smooth. Transfer to serving bowl, cover with plastic wrap, and refrigerate. Or serve immediately with chips or vegetables. Yield: 2 to 3 servings.

Note: This is a basic guacamole with raw garlic featured because garlic is helpful to Candida patients. You can substitute an equal amount of chopped shallots or onions instead of garlic. Stir chopped, fresh tomatoes and/or minced red onion into guacamole after removing from blender, if desired. Buy second avocado for this recipe, in case first is flavorless. Those allergic to both lemon and lime should add small amount of vitamin C crystals (pure ascorbic acid) to retain green color and provide tangy citrus taste.

Clam Dip or Clam Spread

Ingredients

11 oz. cream cheese, softened (can be 1 8-oz. package plus 1 3-oz. package)
½ large shallot, peeled and finely-minced
½ medium-size clove of garlic, peeled and finely-minced
2 sprigs fresh curly parsley, chopped
4 sprigs fresh dill, coarsely-chopped
1 10-oz. can whole baby clams, with juice

Method

1. Allow cheese to soften for 2 to 3 hours before beginning.
2. In bowl, with fork or spoon, mash all ingredients except clams and juice. Blend well.
3. Open can of clams, drain, and set aside juice. Do not chop clams.
4. Add drained clams to cheese mixture, blending well with spoon. Add clam juice, a little at a time, blending until desired consistency is achieved.
5. To make clam spread to be used with crackers, eliminate juice. Yield: About 1 lb. dip.

Note: Serve with chemical-free potato or tortilla chips.

Baked Stuffed Clams

Ingredients
1 lb. shelled quahogs (very large, hard-shelled clams)
6 large, hard clam shells*
1 large or 2 small shallots, peeled and chopped
4 or 5 sprigs Italian parsley (flat), washed and chopped
⅓ of a medium-size red bell pepper, minced
Extra virgin olive or other oil
Whole wheat matzo crackers, rolled oats, or barley flakes,
    pulverized in blender
Salt to taste (optional)
Ground pepper to taste
Natural juice from quahogs

Method
1. With knife, remove all tough, unchewable parts from quahogs (there are several). Cut quahogs into very small pieces. Grate and grind in batches in blender with shallots.
2. Put quahog mixture into bowl. Add minced parsley, red pepper, and as much matzo, oats, or barley meal as needed to achieve batter-like consistency.
3. Moisten batter with a little oil and quahog juice. Add salt and pepper to taste.
4. Fill clam shells with batter and drizzle a little oil on top. Bake on cookie sheet lined with aluminum foil in 350° oven for 35 minutes or until clams sizzle slightly. Serve hot on plate lined with paper or cloth napkin to absorb heat.
   Yield: 2 servings.
   Note: When finished, blender blade should be cleaned very carefully; clams are stringy and tend to cling to blade, allowing bacteria to accumulate.

---

* You can find clam shells on the beach. You can also look for them in gourmet specialty shops or settle for smaller ones from your local fish market (if available).

Country Paté

Ingredients
1 pat butter
½ lb. chicken livers, washed and drained on paper towels
1 lb. ground pork, including some fat
2 or 3 large shallots, or 3 or 4 scallions, chopped
1 large clove of garlic, minced
1 tablespoon olive or other vegetable oil
1½ teaspoons barley flour or 1 tablespoon rice flour
1 teaspoon fresh lemon juice
4 teaspoons heavy cream
2 teaspoons salt
¼ teaspoon allspice
¼ teaspoon ground pepper
½ bay leaf, crumbled
4 teaspoons pine nuts, untoasted
1 whole bay leaf
Boston (butter) lettuce leaves and fresh parsley for garnish

Method
1. Preheat oven to 350°
2. In skillet, sauté chicken livers in butter until slightly cooked. Chop livers finely, using knife and fork.
3. Put pork in large bowl. Add shallots, garlic, oil, flour, lemon juice, heavy cream, salt, allspice, ground pepper, and crumbled bay leaf. Add chopped livers and pine nuts to this mixture. Mix well with two forks or well washed hands.
4. Turn mixture into 9" x 5" x 3" metal or aluminum foil pan forming loaf and place whole bay leaf on top. Bake in 350° oven for 50 minutes to 1 hour, covered with aluminum foil. Remove foil during last 10 minutes to brown top. Pour off excess fat into container by tilting pan.
5. Cool, chill, and remove loaf from pan before serving. Arrange slices of paté on bed of lettuce leaves surrounded by parsley and garnishes of your choice. Or use as a pre-dinner snack cut in squares and served on yeast-free crackers.
Yield: About 12 slices paté.

Deviled Eggs with Curried Cream

Ingredients
6 hard-boiled large eggs
½ cup heavy cream
¼ teaspoon powdered curry

Method
1. While eggs are still hot, place under cold running tap water and remove shells with water running. When cool, slice horizontally, scoop out yolks, and set aside both yolks and white halves.
2. Put cream and curry in saucepan on very low heat. Simmer for about 10 minutes and let cool.
3. In small bowl, mash yolks with cream. Stuff white halves with yolk mixture. Decorate with chopped red pepper or circles of black olives and minced parsley.
   Yield: 12 deviled eggs.

Note: Flavor of stuffing can be enhanced by adding finely-minced chives, shallots, scallions, celery, black olives, or any combinations of these. You might also want to try mashing egg yolks with chopped fresh dill or basil, using lemon mayonnaise instead of curried cream.

Fried Zucchini Sticks

Ingredients
3 medium-size, very firm zucchini
Salt (optional)
3 egg whites
Crumbs made from pulverizing whole wheat matzo crackers,
    rolled oats, or barley flakes in blender
Vegetable or nut oil for frying

Method
1. Wash zucchini with mild soap and warm water. Rinse with cold water. Dry well with paper towels or tea towel.
2. Cut zucchini into strips, and salt, if allowed. Let strips sit to release water. Then pat with paper towels until very dry.
3. In soup plate, beat egg whites with hand beater until frothy and standing in peaks.

4. Spread thick layer of crumbs of your choice on wax paper or aluminum foil.
5. Dip zucchini sticks in egg whites, shaking off drippings. Then roll in crumbs, again shaking off excess.
6. Heat oil in a skillet until sizzling, but not smoking. Put zucchini sticks in skillet to fry, turning gently until brown on both sides. Drain on paper towels and serve.
Yield: 3 servings.

Candida Pizza

Ingredients
2½ cups Fearn White Rice Baking Mix (or brown rice, if preferred and available)
2 large eggs, slightly beaten
2 tablespoons extra virgin olive, safflower, or sunflower oil
1¾ cups water

Suggestions for Toppings
Canned plum tomatoes or fresh tomatoes
Canned black olives, drained and sliced in rings
Yellow onions, finely-sliced
Scallions, finely-chopped
Bell peppers (green, yellow, or red), chopped or in thin rings
Frozen artichoke hearts, thawed
Fresh mushrooms, raw and sliced
Anchovies, drained of oil
Pork sausage (chemical-free), cooked, well drained of fat, and cut in rings
Mozzarella cheese, sliced or chopped
Ricotta cheese (cow's or goat's)
Canadian baby goat cheese, sliced or chopped
Fresh goat cheese (*chevre frais* or Montrachet)
Fresh garlic, finely-minced
Fresh basil leaves, whole
Fresh or dried oregano
Fresh or dried thyme
Garlic powder
Onion powder
Salt and pepper

Method

1. Preheat oven to 400°
2. With oiled fingers, lightly grease 4 round aluminum foil cake pans measuring approximately 8½" x 1½". These can be found in supermarkets (E*Z Foil makes them). Or use 8" round metal cake pans.
3. Blend baking mix with eggs and oil. Add water and blend again until very smooth.
4. Using large dinner spoon, spread bottoms of foil or metal pans with batter, as thinly as possible.
5. Bake pizza rounds in 400° oven (without topping) for 14 minutes, or until dough acquires slightly tan appearance. Remove pans from oven and let rounds cool in pans for 7 to 8 minutes. Maintain oven heat at 400°.
6. Select items for topping. If using canned tomatoes, cover pizza rounds with drained plum tomatoes, squeezing and breaking them with your fingers, allowing excess juice to go back into can for other use. You need only a small amount of tomato juice on pizzas.
7. Then place black olives, bell peppers, onions, scallions, anchovies, pork sausage, mushrooms, fresh parsley, fresh basil, or whatever toppings you've chosen, on pizza rounds.
8. Gently sprinkle pizza tops with spices, including salt and pepper, if desired. Sprinkle oil *lightly* over entire tops of pizzas by placing forefinger over mouth of oil bottle. Sprinkle oil around edges of pizzas as well.
9. Put prepared pizzas in 400° oven and bake for 20 minutes, placing cheese (if allowed) on top, for approximately last 3 minutes or until melted.

   Yield: 4 8½" round pizzas.

   Note: If allergic to tomatoes, eliminate them and choose from other ingredients on list of suggested toppings. Plain pizza rounds can be made ahead, frozen (tightly sealed with plastic wrap), and used as needed.

MAIN COURSES

Roast Duck

Ingredients
1 4½-lb. frozen or fresh duckling (thawed, if frozen)
Lemon or lime juice (optional)
Salt (optional)

Method
1. Preheat oven to 450°
2. Remove innards from cavity. Cut all fat and skin from flap in neck area. On other end, fold in skin and cut off any clusters of fat.
3. With sharp knife, gently pierce fat parts of duck's breast and wings ½ inch deep, especially where wing and breast come together.
4. Rub lemon and salt on entire outer skin. Place duck on its back on rack in roasting pan. *Do not put water under rack.*
5. Roast in 450° oven for 15 minutes. Lower oven to 350° and turn duck over onto breast side, cooking for additional 15 minutes. Turn duck on back again and cook for another 15 minutes, and finish to cook in same position for a total of 1½ hours. Turning process will simulate rotisserie method of cooking.
   Yield: 3 or 4 servings.
   Note: Calculate approximately 20 minutes per pound on duck of different weight.

Veal Cutlets Alla Milanese

Ingredients
4 thin veal cutlets (prime young veal)
½ cup brown or white rice, or oat flour
¾ cup oat bran or blender-pulverized rolled oats, barley flakes, or whole wheat matzo crackers (or buy malt-free matzo meal)
1 large egg, beaten
Salt (optional)
Extra virgin olive, safflower, walnut, or other oil for sautéing

Lemon or lime quarters and slices
Curly parsley (optional)

Method
1. Drain cutlets by pressing between two paper towels.
2. On flat surface, on top of wax paper or aluminum foil, lay out rice flour and oat bran separately. Salt bran to taste (if allowed). Beat egg in deep dish.
3. Dip each cutlet in rice flour first, shaking off excess. Dip in beaten egg, coating both sides well and shaking off excess. Then coat cutlets evenly on both sides with bran, shaking off extra bran.
4. In non-stick or regular skillet, when oil is hot but not smoking, sauté cutlets for 2 to 3 minutes on each side. Drain on paper towels.
5. Serve immediately with lemon or lime quarters. Decorate platter with lemon and/or lime slices and curly parsley, if you like. Yield: 2 servings.

Stuffed Peppers Divine

Ingredients
6 medium-size bell peppers in red, yellow, and green colors
15 Wasa Lite Rye Crackers (or other yeast-free brand)
½ cup pine nuts
½ bell pepper (preferably red), cored, seeded, and chopped
60 dark raisins, cut in halves
1 3¼-oz. can pitted black olives (medium) or about 30
    medium-size olives, drained and cut in rings
6 or 7 sprigs fresh curly parsley, washed and snipped
½ teaspoon powdered dill
¼ teaspoon garlic powder
¼ teaspoon ground pepper
½ plus ¼ teaspoon salt
½ cup chopped red onion
⅔ cup cubed mozzarella, scamorze, California "goatzarella," or
    Canadian baby goat cheese
¼ cup extra virgin olive, safflower, or walnut oil
Oil of your choice to grease roasting pan and pepper skins
2 tablespoons water to moisten stuffing

Method

1. Prepare peppers for stuffing by washing and drying well. Remove core, membranes, and seeds.
2. Preheat oven to 375°.
3. In large bowl, break rye crackers and crumble well with hands.
4. Add pine nuts, bell pepper, raisins, olives, parsley, dry seasonings, onion, cheese, and oil.
5. With well scrubbed hands and fingernails, toss stuffing, rubbing ingredients together to increase flavor and to moisten them. Sprinkle 2 tablespoons water over mixture to moisten further.
6. Taking each pepper in your hands, rub entire outer surface with oil. Gently fill pepper cavities with stuffing. *Do not pack stuffing down.*
7. Grease 11" x 9" x 2" metal or aluminum foil baking pan with oil. Arrange peppers in pan to prevent them from tumbling over. Bake in 375° oven for 50 minutes. Parts of pepper skins will get brown during cooking process. Don't be tempted to turn peppers over while baking.

Yield: 6 stuffed peppers.

Note: This is a labor-intensive recipe, but a favorite of many people.

Veal Stew A La Crème

Ingredients

5 cups water
5 pieces chicken, either legs or thighs, skinned
2 medium-size yellow onions for stock
7 carrots, peeled
1 inch of a bay leaf
1½ heaping tablespoons chopped fresh dill or 2 teaspoons dried dill weed
1½ lbs. lean veal stew meat, cut in chunks
Salt and pepper
2 tablespoons rice flour or whole wheat flour, or 1 tablespoon barley flour
1 egg yolk, beaten (optional)
Light cream

Method

1. Put water, chicken pieces, onions, 3 carrots, bay leaf, and 1 tablespoon fresh dill or 1 teaspoon dried dill weed in stockpot. When all juices are extracted, remove chicken and vegetables for other use. Skim froth from stock with spoon.
2. Rinse veal chunks and add to stew pot along with salt and pepper to taste.
3. When veal appears tender, add 4 remaining carrots, cut in thick, round slices. Then add remaining fresh dill or dried dill weed.
4. In separate cup, mix flour with small amount of broth. When carrots are both firm and tender, thicken stew by adding flour and broth mixture to stew. If using egg yolk, ladle portion of hot broth into another cup and add yolk, little by little to avoid curdling. Add more broth to yolk mixture and transfer it to stew pot, a little at a time. This is a classic French touch you can incorporate or eliminate.
5. Add cream to taste, heat through, and serve.
   Yield: 6 servings.
   Note: Basic stew can be frozen in containers and yolk and cream added just before serving.

Roast Leg of Lamb with Rosemary and Garlic

Ingredients
1 4½-lb. leg of lamb
6 medium-size cloves of garlic, peeled and cut in halves
3 or 4 sprigs fresh rosemary, washed and dried, or ½ teaspoon
    dried rosemary leaves
2 or 3 medium-size yellow onions (optional)
Oil for rubbing onions
Rice, barley, or whole wheat flour, or potato starch, for
    thickening gravy
Salt (optional)
Meat thermometer

Method
1. Preheat oven to 450°.
2. Remove fell (outer covering) and as much fat as possible. Rub roast with cut sides of garlic cloves. Cut same cloves into

slightly smaller pieces and place them here and there under skin and in crevices of meat. Insert rosemary leaves in same places.

3. Put roast on rack in pan. Rub onions with a little oil and place alongside roast. *Do not put water under rack.* Insert thermometer in fleshy part of leg.
4. Put roast in 450° oven. Immediately turn oven down to 350°. Allow roast to cook 20 minutes per pound, in this case 1½ hours, or until thermometer registers in vicinity of 165°. This should result in juicy, rare to pink roast. Transfer meat to serving platter.
5. To make gravy, remove as much fat as possible from pan drippings. Add flour to drippings in pan and mash to eliminate lumps. Place roasting pan on burner of stove on low heat. Add water in very small amounts, blending until smooth, semi-thick gravy results. Add salt to taste. Serve hot gravy in sauce boat alongside meat and roasted onions.
Yield: About 6 servings.

Note: You can add peeled potatoes, carrots, and parsnips to onions in roasting pan at outset, if you like.

Rock Cornish Hens with Wild Rice Stuffing

Ingredients
2 small rock cornish hens, thawed the night before
Salt and pepper (optional)
2 or 3 cloves of garlic, peeled and cut in halves
Powdered, dried sage or fresh sage leaves, torn in pieces

Method
1. Preheat oven to 350°.
2. Pat hens dry with paper towels. Salt cavities of birds and fill with Wild Rice Stuffing for Poultry (recipe on next page), which you should make before starting on this recipe.
3. Rub hens with cut sides of garlic cloves. Put powdered sage or sage leaves in various places under skins. Salt and pepper birds.
4. Roast in 350° oven for approximately 1½ hours. Serve with low-carbohydrate vegetable.
Yield: 2 stuffed hens (2 servings).

Wild Rice Stuffing for Poultry

Ingredients
½ cup uncooked wild rice (4 oz.)
2 cups water
1 tablespoon vegetable or nut oil
2 medium-size stalks of celery, trimmed, washed, and diced
4 medium-size shallots, peeled and chopped
2 medium-size cloves garlic, peeled and chopped
1 small red bell pepper, cored, seeded, and diced
¼ cup pine nuts, untoasted
3 or 4 sprigs fresh curly parsley, coarsely snipped
Salt and pepper to taste

Method
1. Boil water in saucepan and cook rice to *al dente* (until firm but not mushy) consistency. Drain in colander, rinsing rice with cold water to eliminate gamey taste. Set aside.
2. Heat oil in skillet and sauté celery, shallots, and garlic. When translucent, add bell pepper and sauté briefly. Add pine nuts, rice, parsley, salt, and pepper. Stir together. Sauté another minute to allow rice to absorb flavors of other ingredients.
3. Stuff cornish hens or other poultry with mixture. Or put mixture in bowl, cover with aluminum foil, and let cool. Then place in refrigerator where mixture can stand a day or so before using.
   Yield: Stuffing for 2 cornish hens or 1 average-size duck or chicken.

Roast Chicken with Oatmeal Stuffing

Ingredients
2 cups rolled oats
2 small yellow onions, peeled and finely-diced
⅔ of large red bell pepper, diced
2 stalks celery, well washed and diced
1 clove of garlic, peeled and finely-minced
5 or 6 sprigs of fresh parsley, chopped
¼ teaspoon powdered sage or 6 to 8 dried or fresh sage leaves, snipped

Pinch of mace
Pinch of allspice
Salt and pepper
Garlic powder (optional)
Unrefined vegetable oil
1 4-lb. roasting chicken

Method
1. Preheat oven to 450°.
2. Put all ingredients for stuffing mixture in large bowl and toss. Add salt and pepper to taste.
3. With your hands, blend in a little oil and water, making mixture moist but not wet.
4. Remove giblets from chicken cavity and keep for some other purpose. Cut away chicken fat from opening of chicken cavity.
5. Wash both chicken and cavity. Pat dry with paper towels.
6. Just before roasting, stuff bird by holding it upright and dropping in stuffing, which should loosely fill cavity. *Do not pack stuffing down.*
7. Transfer chicken to roasting pan. Rub skin with oil and sprinkle with salt, pepper, and garlic powder, if desired.
8. Place chicken in 450° oven. Immediately turn heat down to 350°. Roast for approximately 1 hour and 20 minutes. Skin should be brown when chicken is done.
Yield: 5 servings.

Note: Calculate approximately 20 minutes per pound on chicken of different weight. If allergic to oats, use barley flakes (available in health food stores).

Roast Chicken with Rye Cracker Stuffing

Ingredients
5 Wasa Lite Rye Crackers (about 1 cup, crumbled)
½ cup finely-chopped celery
3 scallions (white only), thinly-sliced
½ cup chopped yellow onions, or scallions, or shallots
5 large canned black olives, cut in jumbo pieces
1 tablespoon pine nuts, untoasted
4 sprigs parsley, washed and chopped

½ teaspoon powdered sage
½ teaspoon salt (if allowed)
2 teaspoons safflower or other vegetable oil
Oil for rubbing chicken
Salt and pepper for outer skin (optional)
Garlic powder (optional)
1 4-lb. roasting chicken

Method
1. Preheat oven to 450°.
2. Put all ingredients for stuffing in large bowl and toss.
3. With your hands, moisten mixture with water until moist but not wet.
4. Remove giblets from chicken cavity and keep for other purpose. Cut away hunks of chicken fat from opening of chicken cavity.
5. Wash both chicken and cavity. Pat dry with paper towels.
6. Just before roasting, stuff bird by holding it upright and dropping in stuffing, which should loosely fill cavity. *Do not pack stuffing down.*
7. Place chicken in roasting pan and rub skin with oil. Sprinkle with salt, pepper, and garlic powder, if desired.
8. Place chicken in 450° oven. Immediately turn heat down to 350°. Roast for approximately 1 hour and 20 minutes. Skin should be brown when chicken is done.
   Yield: 5 servings.
   Note: Calculate approximately 20 minutes per pound on chicken of different weight. If allergic to rye, use equivalent amount of whole wheat matzo crackers for stuffing.

Boneless Roast Pork

Ingredients
1 3-lb. boneless, lean pork roast, tied with string
2 medium-size yellow onions, peeled
Ground pepper
Garlic powder
Salt (optional)
4 small cloves of garlic, peeled
Oil

Method
1. Preheat oven to 350°.
2. Grease roasting pan very lightly with oil. Lay pork roast and onions in pan. Sprinkle with pepper, garlic powder, and salt. Insert cloves of garlic in crevices of meat.
3. Cook for 1½ to 2 hours or until meat is brown on outside and cooked through. Pork roast should be juicy but not pink inside.
4. To make gravy, remove fat from dripping. Use barley, rice, whole wheat, or oat flour, or potato starch as thickener.
   Yield: 8 servings.
   Note: You can make roast into whole dinner by placing vegetables (rubbed with oil) such as carrots, parsnips, white turnips, white potatoes, sweet potatoes, zucchini, and other roasting vegetables in roasting pan.

Southern Fried Chicken

Ingredients
⅔ cup unenriched flour such as brown rice, white rice, whole
    wheat, oat, or buckwheat
1 teaspoon salt (optional)
Cow's, goat's, or unsweetened soybean milk
Olive, safflower, sunflower, or walnut oil for frying
1 3-lb. broiler-fryer chicken, cut in pieces patted dry with paper
    towels

Method
1. Mix flour and salt. Spread on flat plate, wax paper, or aluminum foil.
2. Fill approximately ⅓ to ½ of large mixing bowl with milk. Put chicken pieces in bowl to marinate, turning from time to time.
3. Fill large skillet with oil up to 1 inch high and heat until oil is sizzling, but not smoking.
4. Remove chicken pieces from bowl and shake off excess milk. Coat with flour, shaking off excess. Fry in oil until tender and brown all over, turning gently from time to time. Drain on paper towels. Serve hot or cold.
   Yield: 4 servings.

Baked Veal Cutlets with Fresh Sage

Ingredients
½ lb. thinly-sliced young veal cutlets
About ¼ cup white rice, brown rice, oat, or whole wheat flour
6 or 7 large, fresh sage leaves, coarsely snipped
Safflower, olive, sunflower, or other oil
Salt (optional)

Method
1. Preheat oven to 350°.
2. Pat cutlets between paper towels to remove moisture.
3. Spread flour on aluminum foil or wax paper on kitchen counter top. Dip each cutlet in flour, shaking off excess.
4. Grease metal or aluminum foil pan, or glass baking dish with oil. Line bottom with floured cutlets.
5. Snip sage leaves into saucer with clean scissors. Mix with some oil and salt. Place oiled and salted leaves on cutlets. Then sprinkle cutlets with oil by placing finger across opening of oil bottle. Cutlets should be covered with oil but not doused with it.
6. Cover pan or baking dish with foil. Bake in 350° oven for 1 hour. Serve hot.
   Yield: 2 servings.

Sausage Patties

Ingredients
1 lb. ground lean pork
½ teaspoon fennel seeds
¼ teaspoon ground sage
¼ teaspoon dried marjoram
2 or 3 pinches of ground thyme
½ teaspoon salt (optional)
2 or 3 pinches of ground white or black pepper

Method
1. Put pork in mixing bowl. Add seasonings.
2. Mix thoroughly with well washed hands. Form into sausage patties.

3. Broil patties. Or rub skillet with very small amount of vegetable oil and fry patties until brown and cooked through.
Yield: 4 servings.

Note: After thoroughly cooked, drained, and cooled, these can be packaged individually and frozen for future use.

Ground Veal Loaf

Ingredients
1½ lbs. ground veal
½ cup barley flakes or rolled oats
¼ cup chopped red, green, or yellow bell pepper
¼ cup chopped scallions (including green part), shallots, or onions
3 or 4 sprigs fresh curly parsley, washed and snipped
50 dark raisins
¼ cup pine nuts, untoasted
¼ teaspoon ground thyme
¼ teaspoon mace
1 teaspoon salt (optional)
¼ teaspoon ground pepper

Method
1. Preheat oven to 375°.
2. Grease 9" x 5" x 3" metal or aluminum foil loaf pan or glass baking dish with oil.
3. Using hands, mix all ingredients in bowl until well blended. Gently pile into loaf pan or dish. Sprinkle top with salt and thyme.
4. Bake in 375° oven for 55 minutes or until brown. Serve hot or cold.
Yield: 1 loaf.

Note: Add an egg to this recipe, if you like. Cooked and well cooled loaf can be packaged whole or in slices for freezing. Reheat in 350° oven or in microwave. Use for any meal including breakfast.

Lamb Loaf

Ingredients
1½ lbs. ground lean lamb
½ cup rolled oats or barley flakes
½ large red bell pepper, cored, seeded, and diced
½ cup diced yellow onion
¼ cup pine nuts, untoasted
50 dark raisins
4 or 5 sprigs fresh curly parsley, washed and minced
1 tablespoon chopped fresh dill or 1 teaspoon dried dill weed
¼ teaspoon allspice (a generous ¼ teaspoon)
2 tablespoons fresh lemon or lime juice
1 teaspoon salt (optional)
¼ teaspoon ground pepper
1 egg

Method
1. Preheat oven to 375°.
2. With well washed hands, mix ground meat and barley flakes in bowl.
3. Add all other ingredients and blend well.
4. Gently pile into 9" x 5" x 3" metal or aluminum foil loaf pan or glass baking dish. Bake in 375° oven for 45 to 55 minutes or until brown.
Yield: 1 loaf.
Note: Cooked and well cooled loaf can be packaged whole or in slices for freezing. Reheat in 350° oven or in microwave. Use for any meal including breakfast.

Baked Fish and Potato Casserole

Ingredients
Avocado, olive, safflower, or other oil
¾ to 1 lb. firm potatoes, peeled and thinly-sliced
Salt and pepper (optional)
1 lb. flounder (or sole or other fish) filets, washed, wiped dry, and cut into approximately 3 pieces each

1 medium-size yellow onion, peeled and sliced in very thin rings
4 or 5 sprigs fresh curly parsley, washed and chopped
Yeast-free "bread crumbs" (rye crackers, rolled oats, barley
    flakes, or whole wheat matzo crackers, pulverized in blender)

Method
1. Preheat oven to 350°.
2. Grease bottom of glass baking dish with oil. Line bottom with potato slices and season with salt and pepper to taste.
3. Arrange pieces of fish on potatoes. Top with onion rings and parsley. Sprinkle lightly with oil.
4. Add another layer of potatoes, salt, and pepper. Sprinkle "bread crumbs" over potatoes and parsley over crumbs. Make sure crumbs are well covered with oil.
5. Cover baking dish with lid or aluminum foil. Bake in 350° oven for 45 minutes or until fish flakes when lifted with spatula. Serve with salad or with green vegetable such as string beans, zucchini, Brussels sprouts, or broccoli.
Yield: 4 servings.
Note: This is a homey, European-style dish for family.

Zucchini Flower Omelet

Ingredients
6 zucchini flowers (if from your garden, pick in morning when
    blossoms are open)
4 large eggs
1 tablespoon rice, whole wheat, or barley flour
2 tablespoons milk (cow's or goat's)
Extra virgin olive or other oil
Salt (optional)

Method
1. Wash zucchini flowers. Drain well to avoid watering down egg mixture. Cut off hard cores at stem ends. Chop cores finely, and set aside with flowers.
2. In bowl with fork, beat eggs, flour, and milk until lumps of flour have disappeared.
3. Heat oil in non-stick or regular skillet, or omelet pan.
4. Stir zucchini flowers and stem ends into egg mixture until

fully coated and blended. When oil is hot, pour egg mixture into skillet.

5. Cook omelet slowly, first covered (you can use aluminum foil), then uncovered. When eggs are set and brown underneath, fold one side of omelet over. Cook through until omelet acquires cooked but fluffy consistency. Salt top and serve immediately.

Yield: 2 servings.

Note: You can add ricotta, mozzarella, or fresh goat cheese to this; fresh herbs such as parsley, basil, tarragon, or dill would also enhance dish.

Frittata

Ingredients
4 tablespoons unsalted butter
½ cup diced red bell pepper
½ cup slivered zucchini, unpared
½ cup thinly-sliced shallots
5 large eggs and 3 whites
½ cup well drained and chopped fresh spinach
8 fresh basil leaves, well drained and finely-shredded (at last minute)

Method
1. Preheat oven to 350°.
2. Melt 2 tablespoons butter in small skillet and cook bell pepper, zucchini, and shallots over low heat until soft—about 5 minutes.
3. Melt remaining butter in larger skillet (preferably 12-inch, non-stick) over medium heat.
4. Lightly beat eggs in bowl with spinach and basil. Transfer vegetables to larger skillet and cover with egg mixture.
5. Cook slowly on low heat until bottom of omelet is set. Transfer pan to 350° oven for a few minutes (if skillet handle can take oven heat) or cover skillet with aluminum foil and finish cooking on burner until omelet is cooked through.
6. Reverse omelet onto round serving dish so that brown side is up. Serve immediately.

Yield: 4 servings.

Note: If allowed, unfermented melting cheese may be added. Other vegetables such as eggplant, yellow or patty pan squash, scallions, onions, or okra may be substituted, if allergic to vegetables in recipe. A cold frittata makes an excellent picnic dish.

Goat Cheese and Basil Omelet

Ingredients
3 whole eggs
2 egg whites
3 sprigs parsley, washed, dried, and snipped
3 large, healthy, fresh basil leaves, finely-shredded (at last minute)
Butter or vegetable oil
½ cup *chevre frais* or Montrachet (fresh goat cheese), at room temperature
Salt (optional)
Parsley for garnish

Method
1. Beat eggs and whites with fork in bowl until yolks and whites are well blended. Add parsley and basil to eggs.
2. If using metal omelet skillet, heat pan until bottom is hot and add butter. If using non-stick skillet, add butter and then heat. When butter is foamy (but not brown) and covers whole surface of pan, pour in egg mixture. Prick holes when film begins to form.
3. When omelet is set and eggs are medium-cooked, add goat cheese to one side of omelet. Heat for a few minutes and roll one side over with spatula to form turnover. Heat a little longer and roll omelet onto plate. If you like, rub top with more butter. Salt and sprinkle with minced parsley.
   Yield: 2 servings.
   Note: For more than two people, make individual omelets, since large ones usually are not successful. Do not salt omelet until cooked, to avoid watering down egg mixture.

Summer Pasta

Ingredients
8 medium-size cloves of garlic, peeled and cut in halves

8 tablespoons extra virgin olive oil

4 fresh, raw, medium-size, ripe summer tomatoes, peeled or unpeeled

8 sprigs fresh basil, washed and dried

4 or 5 sprigs fresh parsley, washed, dried, and minced

12 to 14 oz. uncooked pasta (medium-size shells, elbows, butterfly pasta, macaroni twists, or something similar)—calculate 3 to 3½ oz. per person

Method

1. Boil water for pasta and keep at low heat until later.
2. In large saucepan on medium heat, sauté garlic in oil until translucent, stirring frequently to avoid browning or burning. Let sit in pan until reaching room temperature.
3. Cut tomatoes in small quarters and add to garlic and oil combination. Shred basil and add with parsley to tomato mixture. Toss well.
4. In pasta pot, bring water to furious boil. Cook pasta to desired tenderness. Drain well and drop hot pasta into saucepan containing tomato mixture, tossing thoroughly. Add salt to taste. If you can eat ricotta cheese and want to enhance dish, add 3 or 4 dollops (at room temperature) and toss with pasta.

Yield: 4 servings.

Note: For maximum results, find best summer tomatoes, very healthy basil, and very green, curly or flat parsley. For larger group, calculate 1 tomato, 2 sprigs basil, and 2 cloves of garlic per person. Among other things, you can add black olives, sautéed onions, and cubes of mozzarella to this dish, which can be a very creative undertaking. Most recipes for summer pasta require marinating tomato mixture for many hours, which I don't find necessary. Recommended as an excellent cold pasta dish for a picnic.

Stir-Fried Chinese Rice Noodles (Chow Mai Fon)

Ingredients
Snow peas
Carrots, peeled and slivered in small pieces
Red or green bell pepper, cored, seeded, and slivered in small
    pieces
1 or 2 scallions (including green part), cut in thin circles
Zucchini, unpared and slivered very thin
3 or 4 pieces fresh ginger root (size of corn kernels), peeled
Walnut, soybean, safflower, or other oil for stir-frying
7 oz. uncooked Chinese rice noodles (called rice sticks or rice
    vermicelli)
Salt (optional)

Method
1. Stir-fry vegetables and ginger with oil in skillet or wok until almost tender.
2. At same time, boil pot of water. Remove pot from burner and place on unheated burner. Add rice noodles to boiled water in pot on unheated burner. Let soak 8 to 10 minutes depending on thickness of noodles. Cover pot during soaking process.
3. Drain noodles in colander and rinse with cold water. When thoroughly drained, put noodles into skillet or wok. Stir-fry with vegetables and ginger root, tossing as you go along, until noodles acquire desired tenderness.
4. Salt to taste. People who don't have Candida may want to add soy sauce.

Yield: 2 servings.

Note: Calculate about 3 to 3½ ounces of noodles per person, and as many vegetables as you like. If you can't handle many carbohydrates, feature vegetables in this recipe.

Rice Noodles with White Clam Sauce

Ingredients
2 medium-size cloves of garlic, peeled and chopped
1 tablespoon extra virgin olive oil
1 5-oz. can whole baby clams, with juice
3 or 4 sprigs fresh parsley, washed and dried
Salt and pepper
1 teaspoon salt (for boiling noodles)
7 oz. oriental rice sticks (look for noodles most resembling
    spaghetti)

Method
1. Boil water in pasta pot.
2. In saucepan, sauté garlic in oil until brown.
3. Wash top of can of clams with warm, soapy water. Rinse and dry well. Open can and pour juice into saucepan containing cooked garlic and oil. Hold clams until later. Add parsley to juice mixture. Add salt and pepper to taste.
4. Simmer clam juice mixture for 5 to 6 minutes and turn off burner. Add clams, salt, and pepper immediately and cover. *Do not cook clams* as they could become rubbery.
5. Add 7 oz. rice sticks and salt to boiling water in pasta pot. When desired tenderness is achieved, drain in colander.
6. Line bottoms of two pasta plates with a few tablespoons of clam sauce. Divide noodles evenly between both dishes and toss with sauce at bottom. Spoon more sauce on top of noodles and sprinkle with chopped fresh parsley. Add more salt, if desired.
Yield: 2 servings.

Basil-Cream Sauce For Pasta

Ingredients
1 cup fresh whole basil leaves, washed, drained, and
   loosely packed
¼ cup extra virgin olive oil, at room temperature
3 medium-size cloves of garlic, peeled and chopped
½ teaspoon salt
⅔ cup whole milk ricotta cheese, at room temperature
2 tablespoons unsalted butter, softened
Pasta of your choice for 3 people (about 11 oz.)

Method
1. Tear apart basil leaves and put in blender jar along with olive
   oil, garlic cloves, and salt. Grate, grind, and blend.
2. Add ricotta and butter, and blend again. Scrape mixture from
   sides of blender jar and put in bowl (ovenproof, if possible).
3. Cook pasta in salted, boiling water and drain well. While still
   very hot, toss pasta in bowl with room temperature basil-cream
   sauce and serve immediately. If delayed in serving, cover bowl
   with aluminum foil and put in 250° oven briefly, to stay warm.
   Yield: 3 servings.

Note: Farfalle (butterfly pasta), shells, or cheese-filled ravioli
are good choices for pasta. Those who don't have Candida can
top pasta with small amount of grated pecorino cheese and
freshly ground pepper.

Basic Chicken Stock

Ingredients
3 lbs. chicken parts, washed
11 cups water
3 medium to large yellow onions, peeled, or 5 to 6 whole
   scallions (if allergic to onions)
1 large stalk celery, washed and cut in two
2 large California-grown carrots, peeled and cut in half
½ dried bay leaf (about 1½" in length)
½ teaspoon ground thyme or dried marjoram (if allergic to
   thyme)
Salt and pepper to taste

Method
1. Wash chicken and put into large boiling pot with water.
2. Add vegetables, seasonings, and salt. Boil gently for approximately 1 hour and 15 minutes or until onions are cooked.
3. When done, remove chicken and vegetables from pot and pour stock into bowl. Cover bowl and refrigerate until fat congeals on top.
4. Remove congealed fat. You can use stock simply as chicken soup, adding skinned and boned chicken meat. Or use it as base for any soup or stew or for cooking vegetables. Other herbs like fresh basil or dill may be added when using as soup base. You may want to strain stock before chilling, which is an added step but worth the trouble.

Yield: Over 2 quarts stock.

Note: If allergic to both onions and scallions, use shallots. If you want garlic flavor, add two medium-size cloves of garlic to above. You can also add a few green beans or one small zucchini for extra flavor. Stock can be made in large quantities and frozen in smaller amounts.

VEGETABLES

Sunchoke Sauté

Ingredients
2 tablespoons plus 1 teaspoon extra virgin olive oil, measured into cup

3 large and 4 small Jerusalem artichokes (sunchokes), unpeeled, well washed, dried, and sliced into thin circles

1 large yellow or red bell pepper, washed, well dried, and cut into pieces (about ½" x ½" squares)

2 or 3 medium-size cloves of garlic, peeled and halved

1 medium-size yellow onion, peeled, and diced into large pieces

Salt to taste (optional)

5 or 6 sprigs of Italian parsley, washed, dried, and coarsely snipped

Method

1. In large skillet, sauté sunchokes and peppers in 1 tablespoon oil.
2. Add garlic and onion after 6 or 7 minutes. Use remaining oil as you proceed, stirring vegetables frequently and transferring them to warm platter as they brown.
3. Salt to taste and sprinkle vegetables with parsley. Serve hot.
   Yield: About 3 servings as side dish.

Patate Oreganate

Ingredients

5 large, firm Idaho baking potatoes, peeled and rinsed
Extra virgin olive oil
¼ to ½ cup blender-pulverized whole wheat matzo, yeast-free rye crackers, rolled oats, or barley flakes
Dried oregano
Dried parsley
Garlic powder
2 medium-size yellow onions, peeled and thinly sliced
Salt and pepper to taste

Method

1. Preheat oven to 400°.
2. Cut peeled potatoes (discarding end pieces) into round slices between ⅛" and ¼" thick.
3. Lightly grease 8" x 8" glass baking dish with oil, using your fingers.
4. Line bottom of plate with potatoes and sprinkle crumbs on top. Dust with small amounts of parsley, oregano, garlic powder, salt, and pepper. Drizzle with oil. Repeat procedure with next layer. Continue layering process until middle of casserole.
5. In middle, put one thin layer of sliced onions on top of potatoes. Add crumbs, seasonings, and oil, and continue layering as before.
6. Cover baking dish with aluminum foil and bake for 45 minutes. Remove foil and bake 10 more minutes or until brown.
   Yield: 6 or 7 servings as side dish.
   Note: For larger group, calculate 1 potato per person.

Greek Garlic and Potato Mixture (Skordalia)

Ingredients
1 lb. baking potatoes, peeled and cut in large pieces
½ teaspoon salt
2 teaspoons finely-minced garlic
1 large egg yolk
7 tablespoons extra virgin olive oil
2 tablespoons fresh lemon or lime juice
Fresh curly parsley, washed and snipped, for garnish

Method
1. Cook potatoes as you would for mashing. Drain and return to pan. Shake pan over moderate heat to dry potatoes. Mash until smooth.
2. Add salt and garlic. Blend well. Beat in egg yolk.
3. Add oil, one tablespoon at a time, making sure each addition is absorbed before adding next.
4. Blend in lemon juice, adding more salt, if you like. Serve in bowl, garnished with parsley, as accompaniment to seafood or other entrée.
Yield: 3 to 4 servings as side dish.

Vegetables Fried in Brown Rice Batter

Ingredients
1 large egg, beaten
1 teaspoon soybean or safflower oil
⅔ plus 1 tablespoon milk (cow's or goat's)
1 cup brown rice flour
¼ teaspoon baking powder
¼ teaspoon onion powder
½ teaspoon salt
¼ teaspoon pepper
Approximately 3 cups washed, dried, and cut-up fresh
    vegetables such as zucchini, yellow summer squash, baby
    eggplant, onions, cauliflower, and broccoli

Method

1. For batter, mix wet and dry ingredients separately. Then combine them.
2. Slice vegetables in ¼ inch rings or, in case of cauliflower and broccoli, in bite size pieces.
3. Dip into batter, shaking off excess. Fry vegetables in non-stick skillet in about ¼ inch oil.
4. Let vegetables fry until brown on one side; then turn over with fork. Oil should be at slow sizzle for maximum results. Batter should be stirred from time to time.
5. Spread paper towels on serving platter and drain vegetables on both sides. Remove towels and serve vegetables hot or at room temperature.
   Yield: 3 cups vegetables.

Baked Tomatoes

Ingredients

Ripe, unwaxed summer tomatoes (one per person, depending on size)
Extra virgin olive or other oil
Oat bran, or blender-pulverized rolled oats, yeast-free rye crackers, barley flakes, or whole wheat matzo crackers
Garlic powder
Salt and pepper
Fresh Italian (flat) or curly parsley, minced

Method

1. Preheat oven to 375°.
2. Sit tomatoes on stem ends and slice off tops. Make criss-crosses into flesh of tomatoes so oil will penetrate. With oiled fingers, rub outer skins of tomatoes until shiny.
3. In small dish, combine oat bran (or other meal) with garlic powder (use powder sparingly), salt, and pepper. Top each tomato with mixture and then with parsley.
4. Place in metal or aluminum foil baking pan. Bake in 375° oven for 30 to 40 minutes or until tomatoes appear cooked through.
   Yield: One tomato per person.
   Note: This can be served hot or cold as appetizer or side dish.

Carrots and Rutabagas

Ingredients
1 medium-size yellow turnip (rutabaga), with wax peeled off
    and washed
4 large carrots, peeled
Butter or vegetable oil
Salt (optional)

Method
1. Fill large pot one-quarter full with water and boil.
2. Cut vegetables into similar size pieces to insure uniformity in cooking time. Add them to pot and boil until tender. Avoid over boiling to maintain nutrients.
3. While vegetables are still hot, drain and mash with butter or vegetable oil. Add salt to taste.
4. Serve with meat, poultry, or seafood entrée.
    Yield: 5 large servings.

Sautéed Parsnips

Ingredients
3 large firm parsnips, peeled
3 large shallots, peeled and cut in rings
1 tablespoon safflower or soybean oil

Method
1. Slice parsnips lengthwise and dice with knife.
2. In skillet, sauté shallots briefly. Add parsnip cubes. Sauté both until parsnips start to soften and have toasty look.
    Yield: 3 servings.
    Note: Calculate one parsnip and one shallot per person if cooking larger quantity.

Squash and Parsnips

Ingredients
1 butternut squash weighing about 1 lb.
4 standard-size parsnips, peeled
Oil of your choice, or butter
Salt (optional)

Method
1. Cut squash in pieces and peel. Cut parsnips in pieces of same size as squash.
2. Boil both vegetables until tender. Mash with oil or butter; salt and serve.
   Yield: 8 generous servings as side dish.

Petite Peas with Fresh Mint

Ingredients
1 tablespoon butter, or safflower or other oil
2 tablespoons chopped red onion
1 10-oz. package Birds Eye Deluxe Tiny Peas (or other petite peas), frozen or thawed
1 tablespoon water
Salt to taste (optional)
7 fresh mint leaves, washed

Method
1. In saucepan, sauté onion in butter or oil.
2. Add peas, water, and salt. Tear mint leaves into mixture. Cover pan and cook slowly to desired tenderness. Stir gently from time to time, to avoid crushing peas.
   Yield: 3 servings as side dish.

SALADS AND SALAD DRESSINGS

Tuna and White Bean Salad

Ingredients
3 tablespoons extra virgin olive, avocado, or other vegetable oil
1 tablespoon freshly squeezed lemon or lime juice
1 6½-oz. can water-pack tuna, drained
2 or 3 sprigs fresh curly parsley, washed and snipped
Salt (optional)
1 16-oz. can Goya Small White Beans
1 tablespoon finely-chopped red onion

Method
1. Measure oil and juice into mixing bowl and beat until emulsified. Add tuna, parsley, and salt to taste and toss until well
   blended.
2. Rinse beans in colander under faucet and drain very well.
3. Add beans and onion to tuna mixture. Toss gently to avoid
   crushing beans. Let marinate in refrigerator for approximately
   3 hours before serving.
   Yield: 5 to 6 servings.
   Note: You may want to add fresh dill or basil and sliced black
olives to this quick salad which is good for buffet or picnic. I
chose Goya Small White Beans because they're free of preservatives and taste good.

Fresh String Beans Vinaigrette

Ingredients
1 lb. fresh firm string beans, washed
⅔ of a medium-size red onion, peeled
Lemon or lime vinaigrette (see recipe)
15 or so fresh basil leaves, washed, drained, and torn (at last
   minute)
Fresh curly parsley, washed, drained, and snipped
Salt to taste (optional)

Method

1. Snap ends of beans and steam whole, in very little water, to *al dente* consistency.
2. Slice onion in *very* thin circles. Cut circles in halves and place at bottom of serving bowl.
3. When cooked, drain beans well. Add to onions while still hot and toss mixture with as much vinaigrette as you like.
4. Add fresh basil, parsley, and salt, tossing vigorously until onions warm slightly. Chill in refrigerator in covered bowl. Serve as accompaniment to cold or hot entrée.
Yield: 4 to 5 servings.

Note: This also works well with fresh dill or mint. Try adding 6½-oz. can drained, water-pack tuna, diced celery, and sliced black olives for a great summer salad.

Green Salad with Citrus and Almond Dressing

Ingredients

Boston (butter) lettuce, watercress, and other leafy greens of your choice (enough for 4 people)
½ cup slivered or chopped almonds
1 tablespoon fresh orange juice
1 teaspoon fresh lemon juice
3 tablespoons extra virgin olive, almond, or walnut oil

Method

1. Wash, drain, and dry greens very well.
2. Toast almonds in pan or aluminum foil plate in 300° oven, watching and turning frequently to avoid drying out or burning. Let cool.
3. Mix juices with oil and beat with fork until emulsified.
4. Just before serving, toss salad with as much dressing as needed to coat greens. Serve on individual plates topped with almonds.
Yield: 4 servings.

Salade Jolie

Ingredients
½ head radicchio
1 bunch arugula
1 large bulb fresh fennel
1 large California-grown carrot, peeled

Method
1. Wash and drain radicchio and arugula in colander. Dry well on paper towels.
2. Wash and dry fennel bulb, setting aside leaves for other purpose. Slice into very thin circles; cut circles into smaller pieces.
3. Slice carrot into very thin rings.
4. Toss vegetables with Lemon or Lime Vinaigrette or with Creamy Italian Dressing (see recipes).
   Yield: 4 servings.
   Note: California carrots have more flavor, but other carrots will do.

Creamy Italian Dressing

Ingredients
15 fresh basil leaves, washed and dried
1 tablespoon freshly squeezed lemon juice
3 tablespoons avocado, extra virgin olive, or walnut oil
⅔ cup Polly-O Old Fashioned Ricotta Cheese or some other
    good whole milk ricotta
Salt to taste (optional)

Method
1. Put all ingredients in blender; chop, grind, and purée until runny quality of salad dressing is achieved.
   Yield: 1 cup salad dressing.
   Note: You can use this for dip with vegetables, or chips, or crackers, if refrigerated; mixture takes on thicker consistency after several hours in refrigerator.
   For dip variation: Add 4 or 5 sprigs of washed, dried, and shredded arugula (with tough part of stems removed) and let mixture marinate in refrigerator for several hours before serving.

Tahini Dressing

Ingredients
3 tablespoons tahini (sesame purée)
2 tablespoons cold water
1 tablespoon fresh lime juice
1 clove of garlic, peeled and halved

Method
1. In small bowl, mix tahini and water. Add lime juice and blend all three.
2. Stir garlic halves into mixture. Cover bowl with plastic wrap and let marinate in refrigerator for at least one hour, turning from time to time. Remove garlic and serve dressing on salad.
   Yield: Over ⅓ cup salad dressing.
   Note: For thinner consistency, add more cold water.

Blender Mayonnaise

Ingredients
1 large egg
2 tablespoons fresh lemon or lime juice
½ teaspoon salt
1 cup minus 2 tablespoons vegetable oil of your choice

Method
1. Put egg, juice, salt, and ¼ cup oil into blender jar. Keep cover on and blend briefly.
2. With blender on, remove feeder cap and pour in remaining oil in thin, slow, steady stream. Turn machine off from time to time and scrape down sides of blender jar with rubber spatula. Pour mixture into bowl and refrigerate. Clean blender blades well.
   Yield: 1 to 1¼ cups mayonnaise.
   Note: You may add fresh herbs such as tarragon, dill, basil, or mint during step one. Shred herbs at last minute to retain flavor and, in case of basil, color as well. Let mixture marinate in refrigerator for at least 3 hours to absorb flavor of herbs. This method is much quicker than recipe called "Homemade Mayonnaise," but the other recipe yields better results. Mayonnaise made at home lasts 6 to 7 days in refrigerator.

Homemade Mayonnaise

Ingredients
3 large egg yolks
1 to 3 teaspoons fresh lemon or lime juice
1½ cups extra virgin olive (preferably), avocado, safflower, or
    other oil
½ teaspoon salt
Fresh herb(s) of your choice (optional)

Method
1. In bowl, beat egg yolks and lemon juice with wire whisk.
2. Add oil very slowly, a little at a time (no more than one tablespoon at one time). Whisk and blend completely after each
   addition, adding salt during process. If mayonnaise isn't pi-
   quant enough, add a little more juice. Chill in refrigerator.
3. You may want to shred fresh chives, dill, basil, or other herbs
   into mixture before refrigerating. If so, let mayonnaise marinate long enough to absorb flavor of herbs.
   Yield: Over 1½ cups mayonnaise.
   Note: Homemade mayonnaise lasts 6 to 7 days in refrigerator.
For real gourmet's delight, add chopped fresh tarragon to homemade mayonnaise and let marinate for several hours. Then toss
with cooked chunks of fresh lobster and serve on Boston (butter)
lettuce leaves with garnishes of your choice. If lobster is too
costly, substitute a can of well drained crab meat.

Tofu Mayonnaise or Tofu Dip

Ingredients
½ lb. soft (not silken) tofu, rinsed and very well drained
4 teaspoons extra virgin olive oil
1 teaspoon freshly squeezed lime or lemon juice
Few sprinkles of salt (optional)

Method
1. Put all four ingredients in blender jar. Chop, grate, and blend
   until very smooth.
   Yield: Over 1 cup mayonnaise.
   Note: To give mayonnaise extra kick, add very small piece of

fresh, peeled ginger root and more salt during blender process.

For dip variation: Put plain tofu mixture (without ginger root) in bowl and mash ripe avocado and fresh dill into it; or try adding water cress and cucumbers, or drained water-pack tuna and parsley, or baby clams and fresh dill.

Lemon or Lime Vinaigrette

Ingredients
2 tablespoons freshly squeezed lemon or lime juice
⅓ cup extra virgin olive or other oil
Salt to taste (optional)

Method
1. Mix all three ingredients in cup and beat with small spoon until completely emulsified. Repeat this just before serving.
   Yield: About ½ cup salad dressing.
   Note: This is basic vinaigrette dressing. You can add fresh parsley and garlic or other fresh herbs such as basil, mint, dill, or tarragon. Chopped red onions, sliced scallions, and grated red bell pepper are other possible additions. Use your imagination. Those allergic to both lemon and lime can use oil, salt, and vitamin C crystals (pure ascorbic acid) which will provide tangy, citrus taste. Vitamin C crystals are also useful as a salt substitute; but use them sparingly.

Garlic-Mint Vinaigrette

Ingredients
1 tablespoon fresh lemon or lime juice
1 tablespoon fresh orange juice
⅓ cup walnut, extra virgin olive, safflower, or avocado oil
12 fresh mint leaves washed, dried, and shredded (at last minute)
1 small clove of garlic, peeled and finely-minced, or cut in three pieces
Salt to taste (optional)

Method

1. Mix juices and oil in cup and beat with small spoon until completely emulsified. Add mint and beat again.
2. If you want to remove garlic before using dressing, cut clove in three, making it easy to lift out. If you like the taste of raw garlic (it's good for Candida), mince and stir garlic in with salt, blending well again. Let dressing marinate in refrigerator for at least 2 hours. Beat again before using.

Yield: About ½ cup salad dressing.

Note: You could use fresh basil, dill, or tarragon, instead of mint here. For stronger herb flavor, let dressing marinate overnight.

Grapefruit Vinaigrette

Ingredients

2 teaspoons fresh grapefruit juice
1 tablespoon extra virgin olive oil
Salt to taste (optional)

Method

1. Mix all ingredients in cup and beat with small spoon until completely emulsified. Repeat this just before serving.

Yield: 2 servings salad dressing.

Note: This is good on salad of plain arugula. If you find dressing too tart, cut it with a little fresh orange juice.

Avocado-Pesto Salad Dressing

Ingredients

⅓ cup fresh basil leaves, washed, dried, and loosely packed
1 small clove of garlic, peeled and chopped
4 tablespoons extra virgin olive, walnut, or other oil
1 tablespoon freshly squeezed lemon or lime juice
1 cup chopped ripe avocado
Salt to taste (optional)

Method

1. Put basil leaves, garlic, oil, and juice into blender jar; chop, grate, and blend.
2. Add avocado and salt and blend to smooth consistency, stopping machine and turning mixture with spoon from time to time.
   Yield: About 1 cup salad dressing.
   Note: Buy second avocado for this recipe in case first one is flavorless.

BREADS, MUFFINS, WAFFLES, AND PANCAKES

Apricot-Walnut Bread

Ingredients
2½ cups Fearn White or Brown Rice Baking Mix
½ teaspoon cinnamon
¼ teaspoon ground cloves
¼ teaspoon salt
1¾ cups milk (cow's or goat's) or water
2 eggs, slightly beaten
2 tablespoons oil of your choice
½ cup mashed ripe banana
2 tablespoons chopped apricots
¼ cup chopped walnuts

Method

1. Preheat oven to 375°.
2. Mix dry and wet ingredients separately. Combine and blend well.
3. Grease 9" x 5" x 3" metal or aluminum foil loaf pan with oil or butter.
4. Pour batter in pan and bake in 375° oven for 1 hour or until brown and cake tester comes out clean. Let cool 10 to 15 minutes before slicing.
   Yield: 1 loaf.

Note: Keep leftover loaf in refrigerator because it contains no preservatives. Bread can be toasted and spread with nut butters or fresh cheeses (if allowed). Good for breakfast or teatime, but be mindful of carbohydrate content. Can be frozen in quarters or slices.

Gladys Vaughan's Banana Bread

Ingredients
2 medium-size very ripe bananas, mashed with fork (⅔ to ¾ cup)
2 large eggs, beaten
⅓ cup walnut, safflower, or soybean oil
½ cup milk (cow's or goat's)
1 tablespoon frozen, unsweetened pineapple juice concentrate, thawed
1 cup stone ground whole wheat flour
1 cup rolled oats
2¼ teaspoons baking powder
1 teaspoon baking soda
½ teaspoon salt (optional)
1 cup coarsely chopped walnuts

Method
1. Preheat oven to 325°.
2. Oil and flour 9" x 5" x 3" metal or aluminum foil loaf pan.
3. In large bowl, add mashed bananas to beaten eggs, oil, milk, and pineapple juice; beat with spoon until creamy.
4. Mix dry ingredients separately. Combine with wet ones and blend well. Stir in nuts and blend well again.
5. Pour mixture into pan. Batter will fill pan close to top but loaf should rise properly. Bake in 325° oven for 55 to 60 minutes or until inserted cake tester comes out clean. Cool 15 minutes before cutting or removing from pan.
   Yield: 1 loaf.

Cranberry-Banana Quickbread

Ingredients
1 large egg
2 tablespoons vegetable or nut oil
⅓ cup (generous ⅓) very ripe mashed banana
⅔ cup water
1 cup Fearn Brown or White Rice Baking Mix
½ teaspoon cinnamon
¼ teaspoon ground ginger
¼ teaspoon allspice or ground cloves
40 fresh cranberries, washed and sliced in halves, or 2 plump,
    moist, pitted prunes, chopped
⅓ cup chopped walnuts (or other nuts if allergic to walnuts)

Method
1. Preheat oven to 400°.
2. Grease 9" x 5" x 3" metal or foil loaf pan with oil or butter.
3. Beat egg and oil together in bowl. Blend banana and water into egg mixture until smooth.
4. Add baking mix and spices and blend until smooth. Stir in sliced cranberries (or prunes) and nuts.
5. Pour batter into loaf pan. Bake in 400° oven for 45 to 47 minutes, or until top is brown and inserted cake tester comes out clean. Yield: 1 loaf.

Apple-Soy Bread (Eggless)

Ingredients
2 cups soy flour
1 cup arrowroot flour (starch)
¼ teaspoon salt (optional)
1 tablespoon baking powder
¼ teaspoon ground cloves
1 teaspoon cinnamon (or nutmeg, if allergic)
2 cups water
3 tablespoons oil of your choice
1 cup peeled, finely-chopped, ripe McIntosh apple or one
    medium-size ripe banana, peeled and mashed
1 cup chopped walnuts or pecans

Method

1. Preheat oven to 325°.
2. Grease 9" x 5" x 3" metal or aluminum foil loaf pan with oil or butter.
3. Mix dry ingredients. Add water and oil. Blend well.
4. Add chopped apple (or banana) and nuts to mixture. Blend again.
5. Pour batter into pan and sprinkle top of loaf with cinnamon or nutmeg. Bake in 325° oven for 55 to 65 minutes or until cake tester comes out clean.

Yield: 1 loaf.

Note: You can slice and use this to make French toast. It freezes well as a loaf or in slices. Arrowroot flour (starch) is sold inexpensively in Chinese supermarkets.

For muffin variation: Grease 12-cup muffin pan (preferably non-stick) with oil or butter. Pour batter into cups and bake in 325° oven for about 40 minutes or until cake tester comes out clean. To make batter sweeter, use unsweetened apple juice in place of some of the water; gauge amount of juice according to your tolerance for fructose.

Rye Fruit Bread (Eggless)

Ingredients

2½ cups *unenriched* rye flour
1 teaspoon salt (scant)
2 teaspoons baking powder
½ teaspoon baking soda
¼ cup bottled unsweetened applesauce (omit, if allergic)
1½ cups water
2 tablespoons oil of your choice
¼ cup dark raisins, rubbed with rye flour to avoid sticking

Method

1. Preheat oven to 350°.
2. Grease 9" x 5" x 3" metal or aluminum foil loaf pan with oil or butter.
3. Mix dry ingredients. Then mix wet ones and combine both mixtures. Stir in floured raisins.

4. Pour batter in pan. Bake in 350° oven for 35 to 40 minutes or until cake tester comes out clean.

Yield: 1 loaf.

Note: Spread with Montrachet (fresh goat cheese), cream cheese, or nut butter for snack. Can also be used as bread at meal.

Buckwheat Bread (Eggless)

Ingredients
2 cups buckwheat flour
1 teaspoon baking powder
½ teaspoon baking soda
½ teaspoon cinnamon (or nutmeg, if allergic)
¼ teaspoon salt (optional)
2½ cups milk (cow's or goat's)
¼ cup soybean, sunflower, or walnut oil
½ cup mashed very ripe banana (or other fruit such as peeled, chopped, red Delicious apple)
½ cup chopped walnuts, pecans, or other nuts

Method
1. Preheat oven to 325°.
2. With oil or butter, grease 8" x 8" glass baking dish very well (this batter sticks).
3. Mix dry ingredients well.
4. Add milk and oil; stir until smooth
5. Blend in banana or other fruit thoroughly. Stir in chopped nuts.
6. Pour batter into baking dish. Bake in 325° oven for approximately 40 minutes or until cake tester comes out clean. Cool 10 to 15 minutes before cutting. If using metal or aluminum foil pan of same dimensions (8" x 8"), increase heat to 350° and cook for same amount of time.

Yield: 12 servings.

For muffin variation: Use same batter. Grease 12-cup muffin pan well with oil or butter. Bake muffins in 350° oven for 40 minutes or until cake tester comes out clean.

Oat Bran Loaf

Ingredients
1 cup oat flour
1¼ cups Mother's Oat Bran, Ener-G Pure Oat Bran, or other
    brand
1 tablespoon baking powder
½ teaspoon salt
¼ teaspoon cinnamon
¼ teaspoon mace
¾ cup fresh orange juice
2 large eggs, beaten
2 tablespoons canola, soybean, or other oil
½ cup mashed ripe banana (slightly more than 1 medium-size
    banana)
½ cup coarsely chopped walnuts

Method
1. Preheat oven to 425°.
2. Lightly oil or butter 9" x 5" x 3" metal or aluminum foil loaf pan.
3. Mix dry ingredients. Mix wet ones and combine both mixtures. Add nuts and blend mixture until dry ingredients are
   sufficiently moistened.
4. Pour batter into pan and bake in 425° oven for approximately
   35 minutes or until inserted cake tester comes out clean. Let
   cool 15 minutes before removing from pan. Cool completely
   before slicing.
   Yield: 1 loaf.

Savory Rice Flour Bread

Ingredients
2½ cups Fearn White Rice Baking Mix
½ teaspoon salt
1¾ cups milk (cow's or goat's) or water
2 large eggs, slightly beaten
2 tablespoons safflower or other oil
½ cup chopped red or yellow onion
2 tablespoons snipped fresh dill or 1 tablespoon dried dill weed
Few pinches of ground black pepper

Method

1. Preheat oven to 400° if using 9" x 5" x 3" metal or aluminum foil loaf pan. If using glass baking dish of same dimensions, preheat oven to 375°.
2. Combine baking mix and salt in large bowl. Blend milk, eggs, and oil together. Add to dry mixture. Stir in onions, dill, and pepper. Blend well.
3. Pour batter into lightly oiled loaf pan or dish. Bake in center of oven for 50 to 55 minutes.
4. After cooling for about ten minutes, transfer from pan to cookie rack. Slice gently with sharp bread knife.

Yield: 1 loaf.

Note: This can be eaten at breakfast, lunch, or dinner. You can toast it and use it for sandwiches. It tastes good when heated in oven or in microwave. For freezing, cool thoroughly, cut in quarters or slices, and seal tightly with plastic wrap.

Corn Bread

Ingredients

1¾ cups yellow cornmeal
¼ cup barley flour
1 tablespoon baking powder
¼ teaspoon salt
1 large egg
3 tablespoons soybean, walnut, sunflower, or other oil
1½ cups unsweetened soybean, cow's, or goat's milk

Method

1. Combine dry ingredients.
2. Beat egg and oil together. Add milk to egg mixture. Combine with dry ingredients.
3. Pour batter into 8" x 8" baking pan. Bake in oven preheated to 400° for 25 minutes or until cake tester comes out clean. Cool 10 minutes before cutting.

Yield: 12 squares cornbread.

Note: This could be used as replacement for yeast bread at meal, depending on how many carbohydrates you can handle.

Banana Muffins

Ingredients
1 cup Fearn Brown Rice Baking Mix
½ teaspoon cinnamon (or nutmeg, if allergic)
1 large egg, beaten
2 tablespoons walnut, sunflower, canola, or other oil
¾ cup water or milk (cow's or goat's)
1 medium-size ripe banana, mashed, or ½ cup peeled,
    finely-chopped McIntosh apple
½ cup coarsely-chopped walnuts or other nuts

Method
1. Preheat oven to 400°.
2. Grease 6-cup muffin tin.
3. Combine baking mix and cinnamon in bowl. Then add beaten egg, oil, and water (or milk).
4. On flat plate, mash banana with fork and add to mixture. Stir in nuts and blend until smooth.
5. Pour batter into muffin cups. Bake in 400° oven for 20 to 25 minutes or until brown and cake tester comes out clean.
   Yield: 6 muffins.
   Note: Fearn Rice Baking Mix is available in health food stores. You can use white rice mix if brown not available. Allergenics, note that Fearn mix contains soy flour and corn-free baking powder.

Pumpkin Muffins

Ingredients
1 cup Fearn Brown or White Rice Baking Mix
½ teaspoon cinnamon
¼ teaspoon ground ginger
¼ teaspoon ground cloves or nutmeg
1 large egg, beaten
2 tablespoons soybean or other oil
⅓ cup canned or fresh pumpkin purée
5½ - 6 oz. natural *unsweetened* apple juice (or white grape juice
    if allergic)
⅓ cup coarsely-chopped walnuts or other nuts

Method

1. Preheat oven to 400°.
2. Lightly oil 6-cup muffin tin (preferably non-stick).
3. Mix dry ingredients together. Mix wet ingredients and combine both mixtures, blending until smooth. Stir in walnuts.
4. Pour batter into muffin cups. Bake in 400° oven for 20 to 22 minutes or until golden brown and cake tester comes out clean.

Yield: 6 muffins.

Note: Apple juice is vastly preferable to white grape juice here. You may want to double recipe and freeze some muffins for future use. If so, wrap muffins individually and seal tightly with plastic wrap.

Wheat-Free English Muffins or Hamburger Buns

Ingredients

2 large eggs, beaten
2 tablespoons safflower or other oil
1¾ cups water
2½ cups Fearn White Rice Baking Mix

Method

1. Preheat oven to 400°.
2. Lightly oil 2 4-cup Yorkshire pudding plaques.
3. Beat eggs and oil together in mixing bowl. Add water and stir. Then add baking mix, blending until smooth.
4. Pour into Yorkshire pudding plaques. Bake in center of oven for approximately 22 minutes or until cake tester comes out clean.

Yield: 8 English muffins.

Note: These can be slit horizontally and toasted. Spread with butter, nut butter, or cream cheese. Use also for sandwiches and hamburgers. They can be individually wrapped and frozen for future use, but don't freeze for longer than a few weeks.

Buckwheat Waffles

Ingredients
2 cups buckwheat flour
1 teaspoon baking powder
½ teaspoon baking soda
2½ cups milk (cow's or goat's)
¼ cup walnut, soybean, or other oil
¼ teaspoon salt (optional)
½ teaspoon cinnamon or nutmeg (optional)

Method
1. Mix all ingredients and blend well. (This is a somewhat sticky batter).
2. Bake according to manufacturer's instructions for waffle iron.
   Yield: About 5 waffles.

Note: Substituting water or fruit juice for milk doesn't work with waffles. *Coat waffle iron with oil, not butter, for cooking.* You may add a small amount of cut-up berries or other fruit and/or finely-chopped nuts to batter, if you like. Top waffles with heated, unsweetened applesauce or cut-up fresh fruit. Apple-Cream Sauce (see recipe) is also recommended as a topping.

To sterilize waffle iron: Use pastry brush to coat hot iron with oil. Let iron remain hot for 10 minutes to eliminate any bacteria from past use. When iron is cool, wipe thoroughly with paper towel.

Rice Flour Waffles

Ingredients
2 cups white rice flour
4½ teaspoons baking powder
2 teaspoons salt (optional)
2 cups milk (cow's or goat's)
2 eggs, beaten
1 tablespoon melted butter or oil of your choice
1 teaspoon cinnamon (optional)

Method

1. Mix flour, baking powder, and salt. Add milk and stir.
2. Add eggs, butter or oil, and cinnamon. Blend thoroughly, using fork to mash out any lumps.
3. Stir batter again and bake waffles according to manufacturer's instructions for waffle iron. If crispy quality desired, allow waffles to brown. Top with fresh fruit, melted butter, or unsweetened applesauce, which can be heated and thinned out with small amount of water. Apple-Cream Sauce (see recipe) is another good topping.
Yield: About 6 waffles.

Variation: For delicious lunch or brunch entrée, omit cinnamon from batter and top waffles with creamed chicken, turkey, lobster, shrimp, crab meat, or tuna (served hot).

Pumpkin Waffles

Ingredients
1 large egg
2 tablespoons vegetable or nut oil
⅓ cup canned or fresh pumpkin purée
½ cup unsweetened apple juice
½ cup water (scant)
1 cup Fearn White or Brown Rice Baking Mix
2 or 3 large pinches each of cinnamon, nutmeg, and ginger
2 pinches of salt (optional)

Method

1. Beat egg and oil together. Add pumpkin purée, apple juice, and water. Stir well.
2. Add baking mix and spices. Blend with spoon until very smooth.
3. Bake waffles according to manufacturer's directions for waffle iron. Top with melted butter or unsweetened applesauce, which can be heated and thinned out with small amount of water. Apple-Cream Sauce (see recipe) is another recommended topping.
Yield: About 3 waffles.

Barley Pancakes or Waffles

Ingredients
1 cup barley flour
2 teaspoons baking powder
½ teaspoon salt
½ teaspoon cinnamon or nutmeg (optional)
1⅓ cups cow's, goat's, or unsweetened soybean milk
1 large egg
1 tablespoon vegetable oil or melted butter

Method
1. Mix dry ingredients in bowl.
2. In separate bowl, mix milk, egg, and oil or butter. Combine both dry and wet mixtures. Blend thoroughly, using fork to mash out any lumps.
3. For pancakes, brush hot griddle with oil and drop two table-spoons (or less) batter onto griddle at a time, using first pancake as test. When batter forms small holes, turn pancake over and brown other side.
4. For waffles, use same batter and bake according to manufacturer's directions for waffle iron. Top pancakes or waffles with cut-up fresh fruit, melted butter, unsweetened applesauce, or puréed fruit. Banana Whipped Cream and Apple-Cream Sauce (see recipes) are other good toppings.
Yield: About 8 pancakes or 3 waffles.

Variation: For delicious lunch or brunch entrée, omit cinnamon from batter and top pancakes or waffles with creamed chicken, turkey, lobster, shrimp, crab meat, or tuna (served hot).

Wheat-Free French Toast

Ingredients
2½ cups Fearn White Rice Baking Mix
½ teaspoon salt
1¾ cups cow's, goat's, or unsweetened soybean milk
2 large eggs, slightly beaten
2 tablespoons oil of your choice
1 egg and additional milk for French toast procedure

Method

1. Preheat oven to 400°, if using 9" x 5" x 3" metal or aluminum foil loaf pan. If using glass baking dish of same dimensions, preheat oven to 375°.
2. Lightly oil loaf pan or dish.
3. Put rice mix and salt in bowl. Blend milk, eggs, and oil together. Add to dry ingredients.
4. Pour into loaf pan or dish. Bake in center of 400° or 375° oven for one hour or until cake tester comes out clean. Let cool for at least 15 minutes before slicing.
5. For French toast, beat an egg with some milk (unsweetened soybean milk is okay here too) until well blended. Dip slices of rice bread into milk batter and sauté in skillet with butter or oil. Top with hot, unsweetened applesauce, hot Apple-Cream Sauce, or sliced or puréed fresh fruit at room temperature. Or top with melted butter only.

Yield: 12 slices rice bread or French toast.

Note: You can take 2 slices of this bread and put some unfermented cheese, like mozzarella, cream cheese, or fresh goat cheese, between slices. Then dip whole sandwich in milk batter and sauté on both sides—a delicious lunch entrée.

Whole Wheat Popovers

Ingredients

1 cup whole grain pastry flour
3 large eggs
1 cup milk (cow's or goat's)
¼ teaspoon salt
1 tablespoon unsalted butter, melted
2 tablespoons unsalted butter

Method

1. Preheat oven to 425°.
2. Oil 6-cup popover pan (preferably) or muffin tin. Preheat pan in oven for two minutes.
3. Mix flour, eggs, milk, salt, and melted butter. Beat for two minutes or until consistency of heavy cream is achieved.
4. Divide remaining 2 tablespoons of unmelted butter into 6 equal pieces and place 1 piece in each cup of popover or muffin pan.

Place pan in oven for about 1 minute or until butter is bubbly.

5. Fill each cup half full with batter (don't overload); place on rack in middle of oven and bake for 20 minutes. Reduce oven heat to 325° and continue baking for another 15 to 20 minutes. Serve immediately with accompaniments such as cream cheese, fresh goat cheese, butter, or puréed fresh fruit.
Yield: 6 popovers.

Flour Substitution Chart for Developing Wheat-Free Recipes

One Cup of Wheat Flour Is Equal To:
1 cup millet meal
1¼ cups rye flour
1 cup corn flour
¾ cup coarse cornmeal
¾ cup plus 2 tablespoons brown or white rice flour
⅞ cup buckwheat flour
⅞ cup amaranth flour
1⅓ cups soybean flour
1⅓ cups oat flour or rolled oats
½ cup barley flour
½ cup arrowroot flour (starch)
½ cup plus 2 tablespoons potato starch (flour)

Thickener Equivalents

As a Thickener, Two Tablespoons of Wheat Flour Are Equal To:
1 tablespoon arrowroot powder (starch or flour)
1 tablespoon potato starch (flour)
1 tablespoon cornstarch
1 tablespoon sweet rice flour
2 tablespoons millet meal
2 tablespoons quick-cooking tapioca

Corn-Free Baking Powder

Ingredients
3 tablespoons cream of tartar
3 tablespoons arrowroot powder
3 tablespoons baking soda

Method
1. Mix all ingredients thoroughly.
2. Store in kitchen closet in jar with tight cover. Use as you would any commercial double-acting baking powder. Make up fresh batch every couple of months to make sure powder is still effective.
   Yield: ½ cup plus.
   Note: You can use potato starch in place of arrowroot powder.

DESSERTS

Banana Ball Cookies

Ingredients
2½ medium to large size very ripe bananas
1 large egg, beaten
½ cup walnut, safflower, canola, or other oil
1¾ cups barley flakes (if unavailable, use rolled oats)
¾ cup barley flour
1 teaspoon salt (optional)
¾ teaspoon cinnamon
¼ teaspoon mace or nutmeg
½ cup coarsely-chopped walnuts

Method
1. Preheat oven to 400°.
2. With fork, mash bananas on plate. Transfer to mixing bowl.
3. Add beaten egg and oil. Mix well. Add dry ingredients and blend well. Stir in walnuts.
4. Taking batter into your hands, form balls smaller than golf balls. Place on lightly oiled metal or aluminum foil cookie sheet, about 1 to 2 inches apart.
5. Bake in 400° oven for approximately 15 minutes or until golden brown.
   Yield: About 30 cookies.
   Note: If necessary, dough can be prepared ahead and refrigerated overnight. Bake cookies for additional 2 or 3 minutes if using cold dough.

Oatmeal Cookies

Ingredients
1 cup rolled oats
½ cup barley flour
⅓ cup roasted buckwheat groats
½ teaspoon baking soda
½ teaspoon salt
½ teaspoon nutmeg

½ teaspoon allspice
1 large egg, beaten
½ cup (1 stick) unsalted butter, softened
⅓ cup mashed, very ripe banana
½ cup chopped walnuts or other nuts (optional)

Method
1. Preheat oven to 375°.
2. Mix dry ingredients. Stir in beaten egg.
3. Add butter, banana, and nuts. Mix until well blended.
4. Shape dough into long cylinder. Cut into ¼ to ½ inch round slices.
5. Place slices on ungreased cookie sheet and bake in 375° oven for 13 to 16 minutes.
Yield: About 12 cookies.

Note: A good technique for this is to wrap cylinder of dough in plastic wrap, seal tightly, and freeze. When solid, cut into round slices. Bake in same fashion, but for a longer time. Dough will last several weeks in freezer.

Orange-Pecan Birthday Cake

Ingredients
2½ cups oat flour
1 teaspoon baking soda
1 teaspoon baking powder
½ teaspoon cinnamon
3 large eggs
½ cup (1 stick) salted or unsalted butter
1 cup fresh orange juice, at room temperature
1 cup chopped pecans or other nuts

Method
1. Preheat oven to 325°.
2. Grease 8" x 8" square or 8" round metal or aluminum foil pan with butter or oil.
3. Mix dry ingredients in bowl. In separate bowl, beat eggs and softened butter. Add orange juice to egg mixture and blend well.
4. Combine wet and dry ingredients. Mix well with spoon. Stir in chopped nuts.

5. Pour batter in pan. Bake in 325° oven for 50 minutes, or until top is brown and inserted cake tester comes out clean.
Yield: 1 cake.

Note: For birthday cake, double recipe and use two 8" round cake pans, dividing batter evenly between them. When cooked and cool, place cakes on top of each other, frosting in between layers and on top. Banana Whipped Cream (see recipe) or cream cheese blended with well drained, canned unsweetened crushed pineapple make good frostings.

Four O'Clock Tea Cake

Ingredients
2 cups barley flour
2 tablespoons baking powder
½ teaspoon salt
½ teaspoon cinnamon
½ cup butter (1 stick), at room temperature
⅔ cup (generous ⅔) mashed, ripe banana (about 1½ standard-size bananas)
2 large eggs, beaten
1 cup plus 2 tablespoons unsweetened soybean, cow's, or goat's milk
⅔ cup coarsely-chopped walnuts or pecans

Method
1. Take out butter to soften in wrapper, either overnight or 3 hours before beginning.
2. Preheat oven to 350°.
3. Grease 8" x 8" metal or aluminum foil pan with butter.
4. Mix dry ingredients in bowl.
5. In separate bowl, cream butter and banana together. Add eggs and milk to banana mixture. Combine wet and dry mixtures. Stir in nuts and blend well.
6. Pour batter into pan. Bake in 350° oven for approximately 45 minutes or until cake tester comes out clean.
Yield: 1 cake.

Banana Spice Cake

Ingredients
2 cups Fearn White or Brown Rice Baking Mix
½ teaspoon cinnamon (or nutmeg, if allergic)
½ teaspoon ground cloves
2 large eggs
4 tablespoons sunflower, walnut, or other oil
1½ cups cow's, goat's, or unsweetened soybean milk
1 large very ripe banana, mashed
⅔ cup chopped walnuts or pecans

Method
1. Preheat oven to 400°.
2. Grease 8" or 9" round metal or aluminum foil cake pan with butter or oil.
3. Mix dry ingredients in bowl.
4. In separate bowl, beat eggs and oil with fork. Add milk and combine wet and dry ingredients.
5. Blend banana in well. Stir in nuts.
6. Pour batter into cake pan. Bake in 400° oven for 35 minutes or until cake tester comes out clean.
   Yield: 1 cake.

Note: If you want to make layered cake for birthday or some other occasion, double recipe and use 2 round pans. Fill and frost with cream cheese blended with well drained, unsweetened crushed pineapple or Banana Whipped Cream (see recipe).

Apricot-Oat Walnut Squares

Ingredients
1 cup rolled oats
3 tablespoons unsweetened pineapple juice
2 large eggs, beaten
2 tablespoons walnut, soybean, safflower, or other oil
1 cup oat flour
2 teaspoons baking powder
¼ teaspoon cinnamon
12 dried apricot halves, finely-chopped
1 cup coarsely-chopped walnuts

Method
1. Preheat oven to 350°.
2. Lightly oil or butter 8" x 8" square metal or aluminum foil pan.
3. Mix rolled oats and pineapple juice in bowl. Blend oil with beaten eggs and combine with rolled oats mixture.
4. Add flour, baking powder, and cinnamon. Blend thoroughly. Stir in apricots and walnuts.
5. Pour batter in pan. Bake in 350° oven for 25 to 30 minutes or until cake tester comes out clean. Cool 10 minutes and cut into 9 squares. Serve hot or at room temperature with tea, or as dessert after meal.
   Yield: 9 squares.

Whole Wheat Flour Pie Crust

Ingredients
1 cup whole wheat pastry flour
4 tablespoons soybean, safflower, sunflower, or walnut oil
3 tablespoons cold water

Method
1. Preheat oven to 350°.
2. Mix all ingredients with hands. Form into ball.
3. With rolling pin, roll out dough between wax paper. Place in 9" aluminum foil or glass pie plate and flute edge.
4. Prick bottom and sides of crust with fork and bake in 350° oven for 10 to 15 minutes or until brown.
   Yield: 1 9" pie crust.
   Note: 8¾" aluminum foil pie plate found in some supermarkets can also be used.

Barley Flour Pie Crust

Ingredients
4 tablespoons safflower, soybean, or sunflower oil
5 tablespoons plus 1 teaspoon cold water (more or less)
½ teaspoon salt (optional)
1½ cups barley flour
1 teaspoon baking powder

Method
1. Preheat oven to 450°.
2. In large bowl with spoon, beat first 3 ingredients until emulsified. Mix flour and baking powder together. Add slowly to liquid mixture until crumbly consistency results.
3. Work mixture into ball and, with rolling pin, roll out dough as well as you can.
4. With your hands, press pieces of dough into sides and bottom of 9" aluminum foil or glass pie plate. Prick bottom and sides of crust with fork and bake in 450° oven for 12 to 18 minutes or until brown.

Yield: 1 9" pie crust.

Note: 8¾" aluminum foil pie plate found in some supermarkets can also be used.

White Rice Flour Pie Crust

Ingredients
½ cup (1 stick) salted or unsalted butter, slightly softened
1¼ cups Ener-G Rice Mix
4 tablespoons cold water

Method
1. Preheat oven to 400°.
2. Using knife, cut butter into baking mix until crumbly. Add water and work with hands until ball of soft pastry dough is formed.
3. Break apart ball and place pieces of dough in 9" aluminum foil or glass pie plate. Press dough into sides and bottom of pie plate with your fingers. With fork, flute edges and prick bottom and sides of crust.
4. Bake in 400° oven for 12 to 16 minutes. Open oven and check crust after 12 minutes to see if crust is done.

Yield: 1 9" pie crust.

Note: 8¾" aluminum foil pie plate found in some supermarkets can also be used.

Summer Fruit Pie

Ingredients
½ cup (1 stick) salted or unsalted butter, slightly softened
2 cups Ener-G Wheat-Free Oat Mix
7 to 8 tablespoons cold water
Fresh summer fruit using combination of any of: peaches,
    nectarines, strawberries, blueberries, raspberries, cherries,
    kiwi, pineapple, and bananas that are washed, dried, peeled,
    pitted, cored, and sliced (as the case may be)
Banana Whipped Cream (see recipe)

Method
1. Preheat oven to 400°.
2. Cut butter into baking mix, using knife; add all or most of water. Work dough with hands until ball of soft pastry dough is formed.
3. Divide dough into 2 equal parts. With rolling pin, roll out both halves as best you can. With your hands, pick up pastry in pieces and press into bottoms and sides of each of two 9" aluminum foil pie pans or glass pie plates. With fork, flute edges and prick bottoms and sides of crusts.
4. Bake in 400° oven for 12 to 17 minutes, checking from time to time to see if crusts have browned. Let crusts cool thoroughly and package one to freeze for future use.
5. Just prior to serving, line bottom of remaining crust with summer fruit. Cover with Banana Whipped Cream and add more fruit. Top again with cream and decorate with strawberry halves and/or blueberries as well as fresh mint leaves (if available).
Yield: 1 pie and 1 extra pie crust.
Note: Toasted almonds or pecans can be tossed with filling.

Tofu Gelatin Pie

Ingredients
⅓ cup fresh orange juice
1 envelope powdered Knox Unflavored Gelatin
⅔ cup fresh orange juice
⅔ cup chopped, very ripe banana

6 large very ripe fresh strawberries, washed, dried, and trimmed
of any rot and tart white area near stems

1 lb. soft tofu, rinsed, well drained on paper towels, and
chopped

1 pre-baked pie crust of your choice (see pie crust recipes).

Method
1. In bowl, mix ⅓ cup fresh orange juice with gelatin. Stir well.
2. Then heat ⅔ cup fresh orange juice and add to bowl, stirring constantly until gelatin is completely dissolved. Set aside to cool.
3. Transfer cool gelatin mixture to blender jar. Add banana, strawberries, and tofu (a little of each at a time) chopping and blending after each addition.
4. Pour mixture into pastry crust. Chill pie in refrigerator, uncovered, for at least 4 hours.

Yield: 1 pie.

Note: Possible toppings for pie might be Banana Whipped Cream (see recipe) or fresh goat cheese (or cream cheese) whipped with ripe banana and chopped fresh strawberries or blended with well drained, canned unsweetened crushed pineapple. You can eliminate pie crust and serve chilled tofu gelatin mixture in bowls as a dessert pudding with same toppings mentioned above.

Banana Whipped Cream

Ingredients
½ pint (8 oz.) heavy cream
⅔ medium-size ripe banana

Method
1. Pour cream into blender jar and whip until approximately one third of way into whipping process.
2. Cut banana into thin slices and place in blender jar. Whip cream and bananas to consistency of normal whipped cream. Be careful not to overwhip and remember that using too much banana can result in watered-down cream. Making this cream correctly will become second nature after a while.

Note: Makes good topping for desserts. If allergic to bananas, whip cream with peeled ripe peach or nectarine.

Blueberry Ecstasy

Ingredients
⅓ cup pine nuts
1 standard-size box blueberries, picked over, washed, and
      drained on paper towels
1 recipe of Banana Whipped Cream

Method
1. Preheat oven to 300°.
2. Toast pine nuts in oven, turning and watching frequently to avoid burning (a very short process). Let nuts cool.
3. In 4 individual dessert bowls, toss blueberries, Banana Whipped Cream, and pine nuts. Garnish with more blueberries or a fresh cherry and a fresh mint leaf.
   Yield: 4 servings.
   Note: Other fresh fruit can be substituted for blueberries.

Whole Wheat Cream Puffs

Ingredients
1 cup boiling water
½ cup salted or unsalted butter
1 cup whole grain (wheat) pastry flour
4 large eggs
Oil for baking sheet

Method
1. Preheat oven to 400°.
2. Boil water and butter together in saucepan. Add flour all at once and stir until mixture leaves sides of pan. Remove from heat. Cool 5 minutes. Thoroughly stir in one *unbeaten* egg at a time.
3. Grease cookie sheet very lightly with oiled fingers. Drop batter in rounded tablespoons on sheet, leaving 2 inches distance between each mound.
4. Bake in 400° oven for 30 minutes. Turn off oven and let puffs sit for another 10 minutes before removing from oven. *Do not open oven during first 30 minutes because puffs will collapse.* When cool, slice off tops of puffs (about one-half way down).

Fill with desired filling *just before serving.*

Yield: 10 to 12 puffs.

Note: Filling puffs too far in advance of serving can result in soggy texture. Cream cheese mashed with well drained, unsweetened crushed pineapple or Banana Whipped Cream (see recipe) with fresh fruit are suggestions for fillings. You could also serve puffs with hot savory fillings such as creamed chicken, lobster, shrimp, or crab meat, any of which would make fine lunch or brunch entrée.

Crème A L'Orange

Ingredients
1 lemon
½ cup (1 stick) melted, unsalted butter
5 large eggs
⅔ cup fresh orange juice
1 tablespoon oat flour (not rolled oats) (or whole wheat flour if
   allergic)

Method
1. Wash whole lemon with warm water and mild soap. Rinse well and dry with towel. With sharp paring knife, cut off 2 2" strips of lemon peel and set strips aside.
2. On medium heat, melt butter in saucepan and set aside.
3. Put eggs, orange juice, and lemon peel in blender jar. With cover on, blend until smooth, turning machine off and on a few times. Add melted butter, a little at a time, blending after each addition, until thoroughly mixed.
4. Pour mixture into saucepan (preferably heavy pan) and cook on medium heat for 8 to 10 minutes. Stir constantly with spoon (preferably wooden) until mixture bubbles and thickens. You should see curdling effect in eggs at this point.
5. Take saucepan away from burner and add flour, beating mixture with spoon until flour is thoroughly absorbed. Pour mixture back into blender. Blend briefly, until consistency of very smooth cream is achieved.
6. Pour cream in serving bowl and serve hot on cakes, quickbreads, and other desserts. Or cover with aluminum foil with holes punched in it and let cool. When cool, place cream

in refrigerator to chill for several hours. Serve chilled on cut-up fruit or on other desserts, topped with toasted or untoasted nuts, if desired.

Apple-Cream Sauce

Ingredients
¼ cup heavy cream
2 tablespoons bottled unsweetened applesauce
2 pinches of cinnamon (or nutmeg, if allergic)

Method
1. On medium heat using saucepan, heat cream, applesauce, and spice. Stir and heat through (do not boil). Serve hot. If thicker consistency preferred, add small amount of rice flour or flour of your choice.

Note: Applesauce gives this a lumpy consistency which is okay. Use freshly purchased spice, if possible (to avoid any mold). Serve hot over Hot Pumpkin Pudding, pancakes, waffles, French toast, quickbreads, cakes, or anything you like.

Hot Pumpkin Pudding

Ingredients
1 large egg
1 cup canned pumpkin purée (sometimes labeled "squash" on can)
¼ cup milk (cow's or goat's)
2 teaspoons butter, melted
½ cup unsweetened applesauce
½ cup unsweetened apple juice
1½ teaspoons arrowroot powder
¼ teaspoon cinnamon
¼ teaspoon ground ginger
¼ teaspoon nutmeg
Few pinches of salt

Method

1. Beat egg in mixing bowl. Add pumpkin, milk, butter, and applesauce. Stir together.
2. Add apple juice, arrowroot powder, and spices. Blend with spoon until very smooth.
3. Pour into lightly buttered or oiled small baking dish. Bake for 15 minutes in oven preheated to 450°. Lower heat to 350° and bake for additional 50 minutes. Serve hot with Apple-Cream Sauce.
   Yield: About 3 servings.

Pineapple Rice Pudding

Ingredients

½ cup pineapple juice reserved from 8-oz. can unsweetened crushed pineapple
½ cup unsweetened crushed pineapple (from 8-oz. can above), well drained
3 large eggs, slightly beaten
1½ cups milk (cow's or goat's)
1 cup cooked white or brown rice
¼ teaspoon nutmeg
Butter for top

Method

1. Preheat oven to 325°.
2. Beat juice, pineapple, and eggs in bowl.
3. In saucepan, scald milk (simmer slowly until it begins to bubble).
4. Add scalded milk to egg mixture, a little at a time to avoid curdling. Add cooked rice and nutmeg. Stir well.
5. Lightly grease 1-quart glass casserole baking dish with butter.
6. Pour mixture into casserole dish. Sprinkle top with nutmeg and dot with small pieces of butter.
7. Put baking dish in pan containing few inches of boiling water. Place in 325° oven for 55 to 65 minutes. Store any leftover pudding in refrigerator.
   Yield: 6 servings.

Natural Jello

Ingredients
⅓ cup cold water
1 envelope Knox Unflavored Gelatin
1⅔ cups bottled Welch's grape juice (dark juice from Concord grapes)
1 cup sliced banana or other cut-up fruit (with exception of fresh or frozen pineapple)

Method
1. Mix gelatin and water in bottom of 3-cup (or larger) serving bowl.
2. Shake juice well in bottle before measuring. Cook juice in saucepan on low boil for 10 minutes to kill any mold. Stir frequently. (If not particularly sensitive to mold on grapes, heat juice to boiling point, rather than cooking for 10 minutes.)
3. While still hot, remove juice from stove and pour into serving bowl. Stir until gelatin is completely dissolved.
4. Chill jello in refrigerator (covered with plastic wrap) until it acquires consistency of egg whites. Stir in cut-up fruit and chill until very firm.
   Yield: About 5 servings.
   Note: Eat in moderation because natural jello is high in fructose. Can be made with other juices as well. If using fresh juice such as orange, grapefruit, or apple, heat juice only until hot. Add to gelatin mixture in bowl, stir until gelatin is completely dissolved, and proceed with recipe.

Roasted Chestnuts

Ingredients
Raw plump chestnuts in shells

Method
1. Preheat oven to 425°.
2. With sharp paring knife, carve criss-crosses into "bellies" of chestnuts to keep from exploding in oven.
3. Place in aluminum foil pie plate. Bake in 425° oven for 15 to 20 minutes or until cooked to mealy consistency.

4. Serve hot chestnuts with napkins to avoid burning fingers when removing shells.

Note: Calculate 6 to 8 chestnuts per person. A nice snack for watching television on a cold night. Serve with herb tea.

BEVERAGES

Pink Champagne

Ingredients
1 cup seeded and chopped red watermelon
4 teaspoons freshly squeezed lime juice (or lemon, if allergic)

Method
1. Purée watermelon and juice in blender.
2. In large stem glass (about an 8-oz.glass), spoon 4 tablespoons of watermelon purée. Fill glass to top with seltzer or other sparkling water. To reduce sweetness, use less purée.
Yield: 3 or 4 drinks.

Strawberry Frappé

Ingredients
¾ cup fresh grapefruit juice
¼ cup fresh orange juice
2 teaspoons fresh lime juice
1 standard-size ripe banana, peeled and chopped
6 large strawberries, washed, hulled, trimmed of any rot
    and tart white area near stem, and chopped (about 1 cup)

Method
1. Put all juices into blender jar with banana. Chop, grate, and blend until smooth.
2. Add strawberries. Blend again and liquefy. Serve in stem glasses.
Yield: 2 drinks.
Note: A tart pick-me-up or "cocktail" before dinner.

Pink Daffodil

Ingredients
1 cup peeled, cored, and diced fresh pineapple (cold)
1 cup peeled and diced fresh peach (cold)

Method
1. Put fruit into blender jar. Chop, grind, and blend, stopping blender from time to time to maneuver chunks of fruit to area of blade.
2. Purée until smooth and serve in stem glasses.
   Yield: 1½ cups or 3 small drinks.
   Note: Can be diluted with cow's, goat's, or unsweetened soybean milk or seltzer water. For me, stirring in some cold light cream (to taste), just before serving, is a wonderful treat.

Tofu-Lime Cocktail

Ingredients
¾ cup tofu, rinsed, drained, and chopped (cold)
1 cup fresh orange juice (cold)
1 tablespoon fresh lime juice
½ medium-size ripe banana, peeled and chopped
1 standard-size ripe kiwi fruit, peeled, and chopped (cold)

Method
1. Put tofu, juices, and banana in blender jar. Chop, grind, and purée.
2. Add kiwi. Chop, grind, and blend until smooth. Serve in stem glasses.
   Yield: 2 or 3 drinks.
   Note: This is a tart and flavorful drink.

Grapefruit-Tofu Drink

Ingredients
1 cup fresh grapefruit juice
1 4-inch hunk ripe banana, sliced
1 standard-size ripe nectarine, peeled and chopped

10 healthy, fresh raspberries (free of rot and mold)
1 cup tofu, rinsed, drained, and chopped (cold)
¼ cup ice cold water (optional)

Method
1. Put juice, banana, nectarine, and raspberries in blender jar. Chop, grind, and blend.
2. Add tofu and cold water. Chop, grind, and frappé until very smooth.
   Yield: 3 or 4 drinks.
   Note: This is less sweet than some other tofu shakes. To increase tartness, eliminate banana.

Mango Velvet

Ingredients
1 cup peeled and chopped super-ripe mango
5 fresh grapefruit segments (preferably pink), with membrane removed
1 cup tofu, rinsed, drained, and chopped (cold)
½ cup ice cold water

Method
1. Put all ingredients in blender jar. Chop, blend, and purée until smooth. Serve in stem glasses.
   Yield: 3 or 4 drinks.
   Note: To reduce sweetness, use less mango.

Blueberry Smoothie

Ingredients
½ cup blueberries, picked over, washed, and drained (chilled)
1 cup peeled, seeded, and chopped red watermelon (chilled)
1 cup tofu, rinsed, drained, and chopped (cold)
Ice cold water (optional)

Method
1. Put blueberries, watermelon, and tofu in blender jar. Chop, grind, and blend until very smooth.

2. Add cold water to make thinner drink, if you like. Serve in stem glasses.
   Yield: 2 or 3 drinks.

Pink Carnation

Ingredients
1 cup peeled, seeded, and diced red watermelon (chilled)
1 large (not very ripe) peach, washed, peeled, and chopped (chilled) (about 1 cup)
1 cup tofu, rinsed, drained, and chopped (cold)
Ice cold water

Method
1. Put watermelon and peach in blender jar. Chop, grind, and blend.
2. Add tofu. Chop, grind, and frappé until very smooth.
3. Dilute with water, if thinner drink desired. Serve in stem glasses.
   Yield: 2 drinks.
   Note: If this has too much fruit sugar for you, use less watermelon and dilute with water.

Pineapple Alexander

Ingredients
1/3 large very ripe banana, sliced
1/2 cup canned unsweetened pineapple juice (cold)
1/2 cup light cream (cold)
1/4 cup cow's or goat's milk (cold)
2 pinches of freshly grated nutmeg

Method
1. Put banana in blender jar with juice. Chop, grate, and purée until smooth.
2. Add other ingredients and blend *very briefly* to prevent cream from whipping. Serve in stem glasses.
   Yield: 2 drinks plus.

Peachy Creamer

Ingredients
3 medium-size fresh ripe peaches, peeled and sliced (chilled)
1 20-oz. can unsweetened crushed pineapple, with juice (chilled)
Cow's, goat's, or soybean milk to taste (cold)

Method
1. Put peaches in blender jar with pineapple and juice. Chop, grate, and blend.
2. Add milk to taste and blend again. Serve in stem glasses.
   Yield: About 6 drinks (depending on amount of milk added).

Strawberry Heaven

Ingredients
2 pieces fresh ginger root (size of two corn kernels), peeled and finely-minced
4 large, sweet, fresh strawberries, hulled, washed, trimmed of any rot, and sliced
½ cup thinly-sliced ripe banana
¼ cup plus 2 tablespoons fresh orange juice (chilled)
½ cup light cream (cold)

Method
1. Put ginger root, strawberries, banana, and orange juice in blender jar. Grate, grind, and thoroughly blend.
2. Add light cream and blend *very briefly* to prevent cream from whipping. Serve in stem glasses.
   Yield: 2 drinks.

Case Histories

Mary

Mary had a skin condition variously described as psoriasis, eczema, and allergic dermatitis. Her rash and the flaking, cracking skin covered more than half her body. Her hands and lower arms, cracking to the point of bleeding and oozing with the least pressure, were the most affected. The condition had caused her to avoid the sun for the past five years; she covered her body completely when outside in the summer, which made it impossible for her to swim or to participate in outdoor activities with her family. All treatment by dermatologists had failed to provide more than partial, temporary relief.

When Mary came to the clinic, her husband had just accepted a new job assignment in Albuquerque, New Mexico. She had two months to improve her condition. She knew that if her problem was this bad when she was living in Connecticut, it would be much worse in a hotter, sunnier climate.

Her doctor suspected that Candida had infected her skin and, possibly, her intestinal tract. Until this was treated, she would continue to have symptoms. The suspicions were confirmed by a blood test and a microscopic examination of skin scrapings, and treatment was started. The treatment she received was both *internal and external*, because not only was the Candida growing on her body's surface, causing her rash, but the toxins created by the immune system's battle in her body were being excreted by her skin, worsening the rash.

After ten days of treatment, the rash began to disappear all over her body. Within six weeks, thickened skin on only a few fingers remained. Three months after she started treatment, her doctor received a picture of her taken next to a swimming pool in her bikini; she was tanned.

Mary must continue to observe some dietary restrictions and take multivitamins daily. Otherwise, she is free to enjoy a normal life. She describes the change as miraculous and her family reports that she is completely cured.

Sandy

For many years, Sandy had felt her energy slipping away. Her job as a freelance graphics designer and artist required her to work very intensely for short periods in order to complete assignments on time. Not only was this task becoming more and more difficult, but she felt her creativity and self esteem suffering as well. Foods that she had become accustomed to including in her diet were causing more and more problems; acne, cramps, and symptoms associated with her menstrual cycle were causing her to lose valuable work time.

She first came to the clinic complaining of water retention and "problem" skin. After examination and discussion, it became apparent that the root of her problems was *Candida albicans*. Within the first two months of treatment, her energy and sleep patterns improved dramatically. Her periods ceased to be troublesome. Her periodic acne was the last symptom to respond to treatment. Today she enjoys a clear, radiant complexion. However, if she strays too far from her diet or pushes herself too hard, she notices a dryness beginning on her cheeks; then she knows that she needs to return to a more restricted regimen for a few days. She recently told her doctor that she can now spend a weekend in Manhattan working three fourteen-hour days and still maintain her energy and complexion—a dramatic change from when she was first seen.

John

This eighteen-month-old boy was diagnosed as suffering from a condition called "failure to thrive." He was small and underweight for his age, and he was a finicky eater who was constantly colicky. His parents noted that the baby was always gassy and that his stools had a smell that resembled stale beer. John had been started on formula early because his mother felt that her milk might not be enough and that it might even be responsible for his condition. He reacted to the usual wheat cereals and cow's milk preparations; he craved fruit and sweets that doting grandparents had given him to "settle him down." In addition, his sleep was disturbed by "bad dreams" that would wake him every hour or two during the night. An evaluation by a local behavioral optometrist mentioned the child's difficulty in performing visual tasks that would be normal for his age. John's parents had sought help from many pediatricians to no avail.

The symptoms pointed very strongly to an overgrowth of *Candida albicans*, so treatment was begun immediately, without the trauma of the usual blood testing. His daily regimen was modified to exclude the most likely allergy-provoking foods, i.e. cow's milk, wheat gluten, and refined corn products. An appropriate calcium and magnesium supplement was prescribed along with a goat's milk-based gruel. He was also given a product designed to normalize the bacteria in his intestine and a supplement to reduce the tenderness in his abdomen.

Soon the baby's pale complexion and his bloated belly were replaced by a healthy, ruddy complexion and a normal abdomen. Although he did lose a few pounds initially, the doctor reassured his parents that this was a normal occurrence associated with the loss of the water that was causing his body to bloat. Within a few months, the smelly stool and the gassiness vanished and John had a significant weight gain. Now, one year later, he is average in height and weight, sleeps through the night, and has the mental and physical skills considered normal for his age.

Mildred

A 55-year-old housewife with a recent history of having "disturbing thoughts," lethargy, and unusual weight gain, Mildred came to us for treatment. After moving into a new house, over the past few years she experienced persistent chest colds in the fall and spring. She complained that she felt her family and friends were acting less friendly toward her. She found it harder and harder to perform her usual marketing and housework; she now had to take an hour-and-a-half nap after breakfast and lunch, from which naps she awoke exhausted and disoriented.

When testing revealed Candida infection, her diet was reviewed and found to be high in simple starches and "junk" foods. She had been eating almost constantly since the onset of the symptoms. Within a week, calcium and magnesium supplements reduced her tiredness; she was able to modify her diet and confine her eating to three meals a day. She required anti-fungal treatment for almost four months. During this time her symptoms improved overall, but flared periodically from time to time.

The flaring recurrences are typical of what is commonly referred to as "die-off," as the Candida is eradicated.

When she was finally stabilized on a good diet and modest nutritional regime, her doctor began to investigate the cause of her seasonal chest colds and found that she was sensitive to some of the building materials and furnishings in her new house. When she and her husband sold the house and moved into an older, drier house with different furnishings, the colds disappeared. Mildred was able to return to a normal life and realized that her friends were still with her.

Joan

Since the depression following the birth of her son (now 16 years old), Joan had been suffering from Hashimoto's thyroiditis (an auto-immune disorder in which the body periodically attacks the thyroid, regarding it as a foreign tissue). She also suffered from chest pains which were diagnosed as pericarditis, an inflammation of the sac surrounding the heart. After repeated attempts to find a way of controlling her problems, she came for evaluation.

Since the doctors at the clinic had seen many cases of auto-immune disease in conjunction with candidiasis, and since Joan had not been tested for candidiasis, we began tests immediately. Joan tested positive for a long-standing Candida infection and she began therapy. The course of her recovery was not without problems, as she needed to be hospitalized on two occasions for her pericarditis. However, Joan has now been well for the past six months. Thyroid tests have remained negative and we are optimistic that in time she may have longer periods between attacks and that she may lead a more normal life.

Jenny

Jenny, referred by her periodontist, suffered from chronic, progressive infection of the gums, which failed to respond to conventional therapy. The dentist was convinced that yeast was responsible, since he had read published clinical studies that showed that many such problems are caused by yeast overgrowth, and he referred her to a naturopath at the clinic.

Jenny's treatment progressed slowly and, with the help of

appropriate periodontal surgery and vigorous cleaning of the gums by both dentist and patient, the progressive infection was cured. Jenny's problem is now under control.

Bill

An artist living in New Jersey, Bill had been complaining of a "dry right eye" for the past nine years. His eye doctor informed him that he had sica syndrome, a condition from which the eye, for various reasons, loses its ability to lubricate itself. He had been using artificial tear preparations and went to the doctor seeking an alternative. A review of his records showed that the eye had never had any pus, discharge, or any other signs of bacterial infection. The continuous dryness and negative cultures of the eye fluid ruled out a viral infection. The next logical suspicion was Candida. After a weak but positive blood test, Bill was treated with an oral anti-fungal medication (Capricin), as well as vitamin E, borage oil, and cod liver oil extract (E.P.A.). Eye drops specially formulated at the clinic, after consultation with a qualified optometrist, were also prescribed. Suddenly, after ten weeks of treatment, his eye began to shed its own tears, and it has continued to do so for the last three years—a truly remarkable case.

Afterword

The usual orientation in medicine, trying to find a "causative organism" or "surgical cure," is not useful in the understanding or management of the Candida Syndrome. *Candida albicans* is, in fact, an organism normally present in about 70% of the healthy population. We need to think of the symptoms associated with this condition as a reflection of an imbalance of the internal environment. Good health is really the maintenance of homeostasis (balance) in the body. The dynamic, healthy interaction between internal and external environments allows a lifestyle free from illness and full of robust vitality.

The Candida Syndrome, also known as Atypical Candidiasis, is really the result of the body's inability to hold back the growth of the Candida organism. The systemic symptoms associated with the disease are caused by toxins secreted as the organism grows. As the Candida organism produces more and more toxins (waste products), the body becomes less and less able to bring itself back into balance. This vicious cycle allows the Candida to overgrow even more. As this continues, bacteria and viruses overgrow as well, increasing the severity of the symptoms.

In the first phase of treatment we use antioxidant vitamins and minerals to stabilize the intestinal lining. High levels of these nutrients may be necessary to accomplish this. Often, this first phase of treatment can be completed in three to seven weeks.

The most important aspect of the diet at this point is the avoidance of those foods to which the individual knows he or she is allergic. If one is not sure of any particular allergies, it makes sense to avoid those foods which generally have the highest degree of allergenicity (likelihood of provoking an allergic reaction). The most frequent offenders are cow's milk, wheat, and corn, in that order. As the treatment regime progresses, other foods will emerge as allergens for that individual. These foods must then be eliminated from the diet. (In the third phase of treatment, after the organism is under control, we will reintroduce those foods, one at a time, to determine whether or not they are true allergies.) In this way, we gradually create the specific diet which will be most helpful in controlling the condition.

It is a good idea to eliminate, along with specific allergens, foods that contain yeast, molds, and products of fermentation. Contrary to what many people believe, these foods do not increase symptoms by increasing the Candida overgrowth. The reason these foods increase Candida symptoms is most likely due to the fact that they compete with the Candida for food and space in the intestinal wall. They actually kill off the Candida, causing what is known as a "Herxheimer reaction" (a release of toxins by the dead Candida organisms). This is "too much, too soon" in the treatment program. (Some of these foods will be useful in the third phase.)

The second phase of treatment involves the use of anti-fungal preparations. It was initially thought by some that Nystatin was the drug of choice in almost all cases of Atypical Candidiasis. We disagree. There was a fundamental error in the research which concluded that Nystatin is a harmless, non-irritating substance which is not absorbed by the bloodstream. In the laboratory tests, animals were seeded with *Candida albicans* shortly before the evaluation began. In most human patients, on the other hand, the Candida had a much longer time to overgrow and become embedded in the intestinal lining. Once the Candida is embedded in the intestinal wall, Nystatin, as well as toxins, can make its way through small breaks in the normally smooth mucous membrane and into the bloodstream.* Thus, in many human patients, a significant amount of the drug does end up in the liver where it may be responsible for creating damage similar to that produced by the Candida itself. We believe that a significant amount of the symptoms found in Candida patients that is attributed to toxins released by the killing off of the organism (Herxheimer reaction) is, in fact, due to the patients' absorption of Nystatin.

There are three compounds of plant origin that have proven to be quite effective in the treatment of Candida. Each of these attacks the condition in its own way without any of the harmful effects of Nystatin.

---

* There is no acceptable evidence, to date, that shows the penetration of large Candida fragments through the intestinal lining. If the live organism, through weakening of the membrane, manages to penetrate and is actually found circulating in the bloodstream, the disease becomes life-threatening and the patient requires hospitalization.

Capricin, a caprylic acid compound, is perhaps the most widely used of the three anti-fungal preparations. It is released, primarily, at the end of the intestinal tract, the terminal ileum and colon, which is the major site of Candida overgrowth in the gastrointestinal tract.

Mycocidin, an undecelinic acid preparation, is the active ingredient in many topical anti-fungal preparations. Having strong anti-fungal properties, Mycocidin is used in cases where the organism is more deeply embedded.

Parecan, the most recent discovery, is an extract from certain South American plants. Unlike Capricin and Mycocidin, Paracan affects the mucous membrane of the intestinal lining, rather than the Candida organism itself. It seems to make the intestinal lining unsuitable for Candida overgrowth.

The anti-fungal phase of treatment should be supervised by a health care practitioner who is skilled in distinguishing between the symptoms of Candida die-off (Herxheimer reaction) and those caused by the overgrowth of the organism itself.

The third and final phase of treatment is the return of homeostasis (balance) to the intestinal environment. We want to hold the naturally occurring Candida in check without the ongoing use of anti-fungal preparations, limiting diets, or overburdening supplement regimes. This is where the individual can begin to reintroduce the foods originally eliminated from the diet, one at a time. If the food causes the symptoms to return, we then have proof that the individual is allergic to that particular food. The good news is that many of the so-called allergies that the patient was experiencing while the yeast was running rampant are found to be only artifacts of Candida overgrowth. He or she was never really allergic to those foods at all! The guiding principle here: Control the allergies and treat the yeast.

Under normal circumstances, the body's intestinal flora (Lactobacillus Acidophilus, for example) keep the Candida organism under control. It is important to reintroduce sizeable quantities of these flora into the intestinal tract. Of the myriad Lactobacillus Acidophilus preparations on the market, two are superior: the DDS-1 strain (developed after much university based research) and Spectra Probiotic (a freeze-dried preparation of many strains of normal flora). By filling the former growth sites of the Candida with normal flora, we are helping the body prevent any new Candida overgrowth.

Our ultimate goal is to increase one's freedom in making life-style and dietary choices. It is not our intention to replace one limitation with another, but rather to free one from the limitations caused by the disease.

Andrew L. Rubman, N.D.

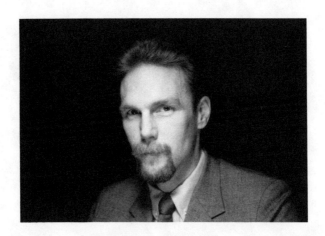

About Doctor Rubman

Andrew L. Rubman, N.D. is Clinic Director of The Southbury Clinic for Traditional Medicines, Southbury, Connecticut. The Clinic is a multi-disciplinary integrated center for wellness. Primary care is offered for all age groups, with referrals to and from all other sectors of the healing arts. A caring environment provided by trained staff affords the patient solutions to health concerns with minimally invasive therapies and modalities. The intake involves a careful review of symptoms and history, with appropriate physical examination and laboratory testing. Upon completion of this initial phase, the consulting physician and the patient decide the most direct, cost-effective approach toward resolution.

Doctor Rubman, who lectures on his fields of expertise to civic, educational, and religious groups, has his N.D. (Doctor of Naturopathic Medicine) degree from the National College of Naturopathic Medicine, Portland, Oregon. His B.S. degree, in human biology and psychology, is from Kansas Newman College. His own emphasis, in his medical practice, is holistic patient-oriented, with a basis in natural therapies and nutrition.

A member of several professional associations, including the Connecticut Society of Naturopathic Physicians (of which he is Vice President) and the American Society of Naturopathic Physicians, Dr. Rubman is also a member of the board of directors of the Huxley Institute for Biosocial Research, Westchester chapter, a Fellow of the International Association for Medical Preventics, and a member of the National Center for Homeopathy. He is state delegate to the American Association of Naturopathic Physicians.

Useful Foreign Language Phrases

The following list of useful words and expressions in Italian, French, Spanish, German, and Greek can be supplemented with a phrase book for travelers. Once again, losing your shyness (if that's a problem) is also recommended. If you're going to countries where languages other than these are spoken, try to find someone to translate the words and expressions on these lists into the relevant language(s).

The underlined vowels in the foreign words on these lists are the ones on which the accent falls. Where a word contains two equally-accented vowels, such as "Alkohol" in German, both vowels are underlined. In cases of single-syllable words, there are underlines only where there might be some ambiguity as to whether or not it's a single-syllable word.

English	French	German	Greek	Italian	Spanish
alcohol	l'alcool	Alkohol	alkool	l'alcool	el alcohol
alcoholic drink	une boisson alcoolisée	alkoholisches Getraenk	alkooleeko poto	una bevanda alcoolica	una bebida alcohólica
non-alcoholic drink	une boisson non-alcoolisée	nicht alkoholisches Getraenk	ohee alkooleeko poto	una bevanda analcoolica	una bebida sin alcohol
allergy	l'allergie	Allergie	alergheea	l'allergia	la alergia
I am allergic to	Je suis allergique à	Ich bin allergisch gegen	eeme alergheekos, alergheekee	Sono allergico(a) a	soy alérgico(a) a
basil	le basilic	Basilienkraut	vasileeko	il basilico	la albahaca
breakfast	le petit déjeuner	Fruehstueck	proino	la colazione	el desayuno
butter	le beurre	Butter	vooteero	il burro	la mantequilla
cheese	le fromage	Kaese	teeree	il formaggio	el queso
cornstarch	l'amidon de maïs	Pflanzenstaerke	kalabokee	l'amido di granturco	el almidón de maíz
cup	une tasse	Tasse	fleedzanee	una tazza	una taza
cup of hot water	une tasse d'eau chaude	Tasse heisses Wasser	ena fleedzanee zesto nehro	una tazza di acqua calda	una taza de agua caliente
pot of hot water	un pot d'eau chaude	Topf mit heissem Wasser	mea tzayera zesto nehro	una teiera con acqua calda	una tetera de agua caliente
dampness	l'humidité	Feuchtigkeit	eegraseea	l'umidità	la humedad
diet	le régime	Diaet	thee-ehta	la dieta	la dieta
I am on a special diet	Je suis un régime special	Ich mache eine spezielle Diaet	eeme se eedeekee thee-ehta	Io seguo una dieta speciale	Yo sigo una dieta especial
dinner	le dîner	Abendessen	theepno	la cena	la cena
dust	la poussière	Staub	skonee	la polvere	el polvo
eggs	des oeufs	Eier	agva	le uova	los huevos
scrambled eggs	des oeufs brouillés	Ruehreier	kteepeeta avga	le uova strapazzate	los huevos revueltos
with butter	au beurre	mit Butter zubereitet	me vooteero	al burro	en mantequilla
with oil	à l'huile	mit Oel zubereitet	me lathee	al olio	en aceite

English	French	German	Greek	Italian	Spanish
fermented	fermenté	gegaert		fermentato	fermentado
unfermented	non-fermenté	ungegaert		non-fermentato	sin fermentar
fresh	frais, fraîche	frisch	fresko	fresco(a)	fresco(a)
fruit	le fruit	Obst	frooto	la frutta	la fruta
fresh fruit salad	une salade de fruits frais	frischer Obstsalat	freska frootosalata	una macedonia di frutta fresca	una ensalada de frutas frescas
without sugar	non-sucrée	ohne Zucker	horeese zakharee	senza zucchero	sin azúcar
flour	la farine	Mehl	alehvree	la farina	la harina
barley	d'orge	Gerstenmehl		d'orzo	de cebada
buckwheat	de sarrasin	Buchweizenmehl	seekalee alehvree	di grano saraceno	de sarraceno
corn	de maïs	Maismehl	kalambokalehvro	di mais	de maíz
rice	de riz	Reismehl	alevroreezo	di riso	de arroz
rye	de seigle	Roggenmehl		di segala	de centeno
soy	de soja	Soyabohnenmehl		di soia	de soya
wheat	de blé	Weizenmehl	seetarehneeo alehvree	di grano	de trigo
goat milk	le lait de chèvre	Ziegenmilch	gala apo katseeka	il latte di capra	la leche de cabra
goat cheese	le fromage de chèvre	Ziegenkaese	teeree apo katseeka	il formaggio di capra	el queso de cabra
fresh goat cheese	le fromage de chèvre frais	frischer Ziegenkaese		il formaggio fresco di capra	el queso fresco de cabra
I would like	Je voudrais	Ich haette gern	parakalo	Vorrei	Quisiera
juice	un jus	Saft	heemos	il succo	el jugo
fresh fruit juice	un jus de fruit frais	frischer Obstsaft	heemos apo freska froota	il succo di frutta fresca	el jugo de fruta fresca
fresh orange juice	un jus d'orange pressée	frischer Orangensaft	heemos apo fresko portokalee	una spremuta d'arancia	el jugo de naranja
fresh grapefruit juice	un jus de pamplemousse pressé	frischer Pampelmusensaft	heemos freskos apo grapefruit	una spremuta di pompelmo	el jugo de toronja
lemon	un citron	Zitrone	leemonee	un limone	el limón

English	French	German	Greek	Italian	Spanish
lime	un citron vert	Limone	lime	un limoncino verde	el limón verde
lunch	le déjeuner	Mittagessen	mehseemehreeano	il pranzo	el almuerzo
milk	le lait	Milch	gala	il latte	la leche
mold	la moississure	Schimmel	mookhla	la muffa	el moho
moldy	moisi(e)	schimmlig	feeseeka trofeema	muffito(a)	mohoso(a)
natural food	les nourritures naturelles	natuerliche Nahrungsmittel	lathee	i cibi naturali	el alimento natural
oil	l'huile	Oel	apo kalambokee	l'olio	el aceite
corn	de maïs	Maisoel	eleolatho	di mais	de maíz
olive	d'olive	Olivenoel	sporeloeo	d'oliva	de oliva
sunflower	de tournesol	Sonnebhumenoel		di girasole	de girasol
soybean	de soja	Soyabohnenoel		di soia	de soya
vegetable	végétale	Pflanzenoel		vegetale	vegetal
on the side	de côté	das Oel separat	to lathee horesta	a parte	al lado
omelet	une omelette	Omelett	omeleta	una omelette, una frittata	una tortilla
with herbs	aux fines herbes	Kraeuteromelett		con prezzemolo	de yerbas
with onions	aux onions	Zwiebelomelett	meh kremeethee	con le cipolle	de cebolla
with spinach	aux épinards	Spinatomelett	meh spanakee	con gli spinaci	de espinaca
made with oil	faite à l'huile	zubereitet mit Oel	meh lathee	fatta con l'olio	preparada con aceite
made with butter	faite au beurre	zubereitet mit Butter	meh vootero	con il burro	preparada con mantequilla
pasta	les pâtes	Nudeln	zeemareeka	la pasta	la pasta
pollution	la pollution	Umweltverschmutzung	moleezmenos aeras	l'inquinamento	la contaminación

English	French	German	Greek	Italian	Spanish
potatoes	les pommes de terre	Kartoffeln	patates	le patate	las patatas, las papas
roasted	rôties	Bratkartoffeln	patates sto foorno	arrostite	asadas
steamed	à la vapeur	gekochte		lesse	al vapor
French fries	les frites	Pommes Frittes	teeganeetes patates	le patate fritte	las patatas fritas
rice	le riz	Reis	reezee	il riso	el arroz
brown	complet	Naturreis		integrale	integral
white	blanc	Polierter		bianco	blanco
salad	une salade	Salat	salata	una insalata	una ensalada
green	verte	Kopfsalat	praseenee	verde	verde
tomato with oil	de tomates à l'huile	Tomatensalat mit Oel	fehtes tomata meh lathee	di pomodori con olio	de tomates con aceite
with lemon and oil	à l'huile et au citron	mit Zitrone und Oel	meh leemonee keh lathee	con olio e limone	con limón y aceite
mixed	mixte	gemischter		mista	mezclada
without dressing	sans assaisonnement	ohne Salatsosse	horese latholehmono	senza condimento	sin aderezo
sauce	la sauce	Sosse	saltsa	la salsa	la salsa
without	sans	ohne	horeese	senza	sin
on the side	avec la sauce de côté	die Sosse separat	teen saltsa horeesta	con salsa a parte	con la salsa al lado
seltzer water	l'eau minérale	Selterswasser	metaleeko nehro	una minerale gassata	el agua mineral
smoke	la fumée	Rauch	kapneezma	il fumo	el humo
smoke bothers me	la fumée me dérange	der Rauch stoert mich	o kaonos meh peerazee	il fumo mi dà fastidio	el humo me molesta
non-smoking section	la section non-fumeurs	Nichtraucher Abteilung, Sektion	mee kapneezehte	la sezione non fumatori	la sección de no fumar
soy sauce	la sauce de soja	Soyasosse		la salsa di soja	la salsa de soya

English	French	German	Greek	Italian	Spanish
sugar	le sucre	Zucker	zakharee	lo zucchero	el azúcar
sugar-free diet	un régime sans sucre	eine zuckerlose Diaet	eeme seh thee-ehta apo zakharee	una dieta senza zucchero	una dieta sin azúcar
vinegar	le vinaigre	Essig	kseethee	l'aceto	el vinagre
Waiter!	Garçon, s'il vous plaît	Bedienung bitte!	Garcon!	Cameriere!	Camerero!
water	l'eau	Wasser	nehro	l'acqua	el agua
with ice	des glaçons	Eiswasser	meh pago	con ghiaccio	con hielo
yeast	la levure	Hefe	maya	il lievito	la levadura
yeast-free	sans levure	ohne Hefe	horeese maya	senza lievito	sin levadura
yeast-free diet	un régime sans levure	Diaet ohne Hefe	thee-ehta horeese maya	una dieta senza lievito	una dieta sin levadura

Bibliography

Barako, Janet L. and Ferrick, Diane M. *Yeast-Free Wheat-Free Sugar Sensitive Cooking, and Feeling Good About It*. Suffield, CT: Healthy Changes, 1984

Barkie, Karen E. *Sweet and Sugar-free*. New York: St. Martin's Press, 1982

Bon Appetit. Los Angeles, CA: Bon Appetit Publishing Corp.

Burros, Marian. "U.S. Food Regulation: Tales From a Twilight Zone." *New York Times* article, June 10, 1987

Chaitow, Leon. *Candida Albicans—Could Yeast Be Your Problem?* Great Britain: Thorsons Publishers Ltd., 1985

Connolly, Pat and Associates of the Price-Pottenger Nutrition Foundation. *The Candida Albicans Yeast-Free Cookbook* New Canaan, CT: Keats Publishing, Inc., 1985

Crook, William G. *The Yeast Connection*. Jackson, TN: Professional Books, 1984

Davis, Adelle. *Let's Eat Right To Keep Fit*. New York: Harcourt Brace Jovanovich, Inc., 1970

DeSchepper, Luc. *The Candida Symptoms, The Causes, The Cure*. Santa Monica, CA: Luc DeSchepper, 1986

Peak Immunity. Santa Monica, CA: Luc DeSchepper, 1989

Gourmet. New York: Condè Nast Publications

Eagle, Robert. *Eating and Allergy*. London, England: Futura Publications Limited, 1979

Hunter, Beatrice Trum. *Additives Book*, revised edition. New Canaan, CT: Keats Publishing, Inc., 1980

Jacobson, Michael F. *Eater's Digest—The Consumer's Factbook of Food Additives*. Garden City, N.Y.: Anchor Books, 1976

Kroker, George F. "Chronic Candidiasis and Allergy," Chapter 49 from *Food Allergy and Intolerance*, edited by J. Brostoff and S. Challacombe. Great Britain: Bailliere Tindall/W.B. Saunders, 1987

Lorenzani, Shirley S. *Candida—A Twentieth Century Disease*. New Canaan, CT: Keats Publishing, Inc., 1986

Ludeman, Kate, and Henderson, Louise, with Basayne, Henry S. *Do-It-Yourself Allergy Analysis Handbook*. New Canaan, CT: Keats Publishing, Inc., 1979

Mandell, Fran Gare. *Dr. Mandell's Allergy-Free Cookbook*. New York: Pocket Books, 1981

Mandell, Marshall, and Scanlon, Lynne Waller. *Dr. Mandell's 5-Day Allergy Relief System*. New York: Pocket Books, 1979

Mindell, Earl. *Earl Mindell's Vitamin Bible*. New York: Warner Books, 1971

Mosby Medical Encyclopedia. New York: Plume/New American Library, 19895

Nonken, Pamela P., and Hirsch, S. Roger. *The Allergy Cookbook Food Buying Guide*. New York: Greenwich House, 1974

Randolph, Theron G., and Moss, Ralph W. *An Alternative Approach To Allergies*. New York: Harper & Row, 1980

Rockwell, Sally. *Coping With Candida Cookbook*. Seattle: Sally Rockwell, 1984

Rombauer, Irma S., and Becker, Marion Rombauer. *Joy of Cooking*. New York: Bobbs-Merrill Company, Inc., 1975

Remington, Dennis W., and Higa, Barbara W. *Back To Health*. Provo, UT: Vitality House International, Inc., 1986

Shattuck, Ruth R. *The Allergy Cookbook*. New York: Signet, 1986

Stevens, Laura J. *The Complete Book of Allergy Control*. New York: Macmillan Publishing Company, 1983

Sullivan, Margaret. *The New Carbohydrate Gram Counter*. New York: Dell Publishing Co., Inc., 1980

Truss, C. Orian. *The Missing Diagnosis*. Birmingham, AL: C. Orian Truss, M.D., 1982

Webster, David. *Acidophilus & Colon Health*, revised edition. Hermosa Beach, CA: R.B. Bernstein, 1984

Wilen, Joan, and Wilen, Lydia. *Chicken Soup & Other Folk Remedies*. New York: Fawcett Columbine, 1984

Wunderlich, Ray C., Jr., and Kalita, Dwight E. *Candida Albicans—How To Fight An Exploding Epidemic of Yeast-Related Diseases*. New Canaan, CT: Keats Publishing, Inc., 1984

Index